Sexy
Challenges

Sexy Challenges

Sacred and Sensual Experiences for Lovers

Rob Alex, M.Msc.

Published by

Inward Oasis

Table of Contents

Introduction

You might have purchased this book because the word SEX is in the title. That is the reason that many people purchase books, either it has sex in the title or the book shows a sexy image on the front. Both of these tactics work and work well. However, now that I have your attention I am going to take you on a ride you might not have suspected. Not only are you going to have the opportunity for some of the most sensual experiences of your life, but you are also going to learn and experience the sacred side of your intimacy with your beloved.

"Sacred?" You might be saying to yourself, "I didn't sign up for that!" Well, before you run away you need to understand that learning this can bring you the most incredible experiences of your sexual life. Bringing the sacred into these sensual experiences is what is going to make your connection to your partner that much closer. Tantra teaches us to cross over into the spiritual aspect of our sexual relations and form these wonderful connections. However, Tantra was developed many, many years ago and I believe it could use some modernization and I want you to have tools that are applicable today. The Kama Sutra is another wonderful tool for connection, but yet again, the world has changed dramatically since the time it was written. What if you could blend them into the intimate play of modern times?

Most of what we hear nowadays is the physical importance of sex. It is good for our bodies; it helps us stay in better shape; it is important for our minds; and it has many other positive benefits from a physical perspective. It feels good after all, and most of us have that knowledge or experience. Could there be more reason for sex than just a physical high?

What if its design was to let couples experience the wonders of the ages? What if it was a way to travel around the Universe metaphysically or to touch and experience the Divine Source that you believe in? Euphoria is medically recognized as a mental and emotional condition in which a person experiences intense feelings of wellbeing, elation, happiness, ecstasy, excitement and joy. To reach this state many people will consume drugs, drink excessively or drop out of normal society. I have to wonder why? If they only understood that they can get this euphoric state from spiritual rituals, meditation, love and yes, you guessed it - orgasm.

That is where the Blended Spirit comes into play. When you are in a committed relationship the energy and Spirit of each partner blends together to form a third spirit or energy. This is the Blended Spirit of the couple. Becoming aware of this connecting of your spirits allows you to understand that feelings are something the two of you share and that includes the sensual pleasure you feel. These feelings are also affecting your blended spirit in an exponential way allowing the two of you to experience transcendence – a piercing the veil between the Earthly dimension and the spiritual dimension. This can take you far beyond physical pleasure and into a calm and peaceful loving spot or perhaps a place of such heightened ecstasy that you simply cannot put it into human words.

Sexual intimacy within a loving relationship builds and strengthens the blended spirit. The more powerful your blended spirit becomes the more you begin to experience things not of this physical world. Orgasms and love are the fuel for this journey. I do want to clarify here that when you create a blended spirit with your love that you do not lose yourself. You remain two individual souls as you create and expand your blended spirit – the relationship's soul.

As you go through this book I not only encourage the two of you to talk about the challenges and how to set them up, but the physical experiences you feel during the challenges, and the climax of the challenge. Talk about them afterwards and express what you witness during the experience. Did your pleasure push you out of your body to another pleasure-filled spot? Did you experience feelings or visions that could only come from someplace other than this world? Converse about the rush of excitement or nervousness you felt as the challenge unfolded.

Sharing your body with your partner to be filled with pleasure can be challenging for some, but once you can reach past those blocks and truly give in to the pleasure you will be amazed at the way your world will change.

This might be a little much for many of you out there to believe. You can take this book and use these Sexy Challenges as purely physical sexual acts. Maybe that is what you feel you and your partner need. However, let me ask you this, if there was a super orgasm that felt ten or a hundred times better than the ones you are having at this point, wouldn't you want an opportunity to experience those? Combining these sensual acts with the sacredness of the love and passion between the two of you and using them to honor your relationship and one another could be like a dam breaking and letting the flood of powerful energetic, orgasmic excitement wash over both of you.

You might doubt these words I speak and feel like there is no better feeling than the ones you are enjoying in your intimacy right now. BUT, what if you are wrong? What if you experience something so wonderful your life will change? *That is what happened to me and I can tell you that my being is filled with a new excitement* and that is what I want to help you find.

Abacus of Love

The abacus is an ancient counting tool used primarily in parts of Asia. It is a simple device usually made up of beads sliding on wires. These devices were found all over the world and in many different forms. So, needless to say the abacus was an important way to keep track of items by counting them. Your abacus is going to help you keep track of the intimate connections that you make as a couple.

Using your primitive abacus you are going to start a process that will go on for as long as you desire. This will create a wonderful work of art or focal point. Your abacus will become a wonderful piece of artwork that will serve as a constant reminder of the passion you share as a couple. The beauty of it is that you can put this masterpiece in plain sight and the only people that know the meaning will be the two of you. Unless, of course, you decide to share this information with others.

This is a beautiful and special way to show off your love and passion for each other that continues to improve each time you make love.

Where to perform:

This challenge can be performed anywhere. The sexual part of the challenge isn't a concern here. The basic part can be done in any part of the house.

What you will need:

This challenge will require some beads and string. Those are pretty much the only things you will need. If you want to hang your work on the wall, you might need a nail or hook. You can change the beads from time to time or you can use anything in place of the beads that you can put a hole in to allow the string to pass through.

How to complete:

This could continue throughout the entire life of your relationship if you choose to do so. Basically, what you are going to do is keep track of each time that the two of you make love to each other. You will do this by adding a bead to the string each and every time you have an intimate encounter. It is that simple. Yet, it keeps going and going and going. Once you start your bead collection of lovemaking, you can tie the end of the string together and hang it over your bed. This will act as a magnet for positive and powerful energy to be collected around your altar of love. Much like the way a dream catcher collects bad dreams this instrument will catch positive energy and love for you to absorb into your relationship.

The beauty of this is that the more and more beads you add to the string the more and more positive energy you can collect into your relationship and life. When you fill a string up completely, you just start a new strand and connect it to the old one in any fashion you can imagine. Or, if you prefer, you could store the filled one in a special place and start a new one. As you can see, over the years your energy collector will start to grow and take on its own life. Can you imagine how large it will be or how many you will have stored away at the time of your 25th anniversary?

There are several different options you can use to enhance this sexy challenge. You can choose different colored beads for each month or year. You could also get special beads for when you make love someplace other than your house such as when you go on vacation. Find a bead from that place and add it to your collection. You could also give your partner a bead for special occasions, like birthdays, holidays or anniversaries. In that situation, your partner gets to choose the time when the bead will be placed on the string. Whatever interesting ideas you come up with to add unique beads to your string, you will now have a symbol of your lasting love always hanging above your bed.

Dirty Girl / Dirty Boy

We all hear the saying "Let's get dirty," which means being bad or doing something wrong. When we refer to someone as being a "dirty girl" or a "dirty boy" it implies that sex is dirty. Why is filth associated with sex and intimacy? This seems so silly to me. Therefore, I am going to take this terminology and run with it a bit in a different direction. For starters, let's be clear - dirt isn't necessarily bad for our bodies. Think about all the mud facials and mud baths people take to invigorate their skin. What if you could get that feeling in your intimacy? That would be amazing!

In this challenge, you are going to use getting dirty as a way to turn you on in a very positive way. This will allow you to touch your partner's body in a very sensual way and yet with a very different sensation. The texture and smoothness or roughness of your partner's body will feel exciting against your hands, and he/she will get cold chills as you change your touch. You likely have never had as good of a time getting dirty as you are about to with this experience.

Where to perform:

I suggest your bedroom and access to a shower once the challenge is completed. Of course, you can do this any place in your house, but make sure you take precautions. I don't want you to get stains in your bedroom, but stains on the floor or furniture are more visible and are harder to explain in the living room than ones in the bedroom.

What you will need:

Get some kind of covering for your bed. It might be a painter's drop cloth or maybe even just an old sheet or blanket you don't mind ruining. This cloth will act as a barrier so that the "dirt" doesn't ruin your good sheets or bed coverings. You can proceed in a couple of ways. One option might be that you go out and look for some amazing skin mud that has vitamins and minerals within the mixture. I ran across Dead Sea Mud that purifies and replenishes your skin. If your budget doesn't allow for that type of a luxury, you could use simple chocolate pudding. It would serve the same purpose just as well. You just won't get the vitamins or minerals the mud offers. Of course, the point isn't so much about what this will do for your skin as the sensation it will create in your body.

Make sure you have soap and a shower easily available for a quick cleanup afterwards. Having towels handy might also be a great idea. Just be sure to use ones that you don't mind getting stains on. As always make sure to have any items you would normally have or use during sex such as condoms, lubrication, and/or toys.

How to complete:

Start by spreading your drop cloth over the area. Once you have the area adequately covered it is time for both of you to strip naked. Make sure your essential mud or pudding is nearby. You are going to want it within reach. Take turns smearing the mud or pudding over each other. There is no rush; take your time and enjoy the way your partner's body feels – slick, silky, cool, etc. Remember this is foreplay, but be cautious too. You do not want to get mud or pudding into places such as the eyes or vagina or anus. This could cause irritation or infection. Focus on the breasts/chest, stomach, back, legs, arms and so forth. You might even consider rubbing it into your partner's hair. Now, you have really become a dirty girl or dirty boy.

Once both partners are covered in mud or pudding, you might even consider being brave enough to take some photos for your private collection. Even if you erase them right away, it will still be fun to see what you look like covered in mud.

Now, you have a couple of options. If you have kept the substance on your body away from the genitals, you could make slippery sliding love to each other. The slickness between the two of your chests could be quite enjoyable. If you have used the pudding option, you can snack a little on your lover. After you both climax, you can whisk yourselves off to the shower. If you are not comfortable or have had the substance move near your genitals, you might want to shower before you make love to each other. This is okay.

Here is one rule for this sexy challenge that I ask you to follow: When showering with your partner you are not allowed to wash yourself. Only your partner can clean you up and vice versa. This way your pleasure can be extended or even heat you up all over again.

If you were able to keep all of your mud or pudding on the drop cloth, then cleanup will be a breeze.

The Date is in the Mail

This challenge is designed for you to have a hand in your next date night with your lover. Avoid another night of speaking to each other and going back and forth with the phrase, "What do you want to do?" You are going to take charge a little and offer some suggestions for the date. Without choosing exactly what will happen you will offer suggestions from what to do during the date to what happens at the end of the date.

What you will need:

Very few things are needed. You will need some paper, a computer with printer, (or you can write it out if you don't have access to a computer and printer), an envelope and a stamp. That is pretty much the extent of the needs.

Where to perform:

You can perform the start of this challenge at your home or anywhere with computer access. The date part and what happens afterwards is up to you.

How to perform:

Sit down and pick three options for each category of the date. The categories being: Time and Date, Dinner Options, Entertainment Options, After Hours Options, and Intimacy Options. Now make a form that lists each one of these categories and the three options for each. Make a little check box beside each one to make it look official. You have placed the ultimate choices of the date in your partner's hands. Yet, you will still not know exactly how it will turn out.

In regards to your options, obviously time and date are when you would like to go on the date or when you are available; dinner options are three restaurants or types of meals you enjoy eating (consider the expense of the meals too); entertainment options can include anything from going to a movie to walking hand-in-hand someplace; after hours options might be going to a coffee house and talking, going to a club to dance, or just returning home for some wine and conversation; intimacy options will depend on where you are in your relationship (a hug, a kiss on the cheek or a night of wild passion and breakfast the next morning). Remember to be sure and give your date three choices for him/her to choose from in each category.

Once you have your form created you need to fold it and place it in the envelope. Then mail it to your love. Even if he/she lives in the same house mail it anyway. This will add a little mystery to your date. Make sure your partner lets you know what time and date he/she chooses with a return letter or some kind of message. Ask him/her not to tell you the other choices he/she made. This will remain a surprise.

This is great not only for new relationships, but for ones that are well established. For partners who have been together a while this can add a little spice and renewed excitement. The beauty of this is your partner will most likely not be able to contain his/her smile when the letter shows up in the mail. It is sure to spark his/her interest especially when selection of the intimacy options comes around.

Body Builders Need Love Too

Okay, so most of us out there are not what we would consider body builders. However, most of us do care what our body looks like. We want to be attractive and healthy. It is not that we want to have enormous muscles like serious body builders have. We just want to look good and feel better.

One of the hardest things to do it seems is start exercising and change our eating. Finding the energy to get moving and make a difference in our bodies seems to be too hard. This is especially true if you haven't exercised or eaten right in quite a while. Here is a little secret for you though – once you start its gets easier as you build your stamina and endurance, and as you start to look and feel better you will want to keep doing it. That should be enough reward in itself, but I want to suggest a special treat for those of you who go to the effort of loving and caring for your body.

This challenge will not only benefit you, but it will benefit your partner as well. Of course, both of you will enjoy the increased sexiness of your toned bodies and the increase in your endurance, but I want to add something extra special.

What you will need:

You will need body oil. It can be baby oil or some wonderful massage oil as long as it makes your skin glisten. You can usually find something that will work at your local discount store. Be certain you purchase a large amount. You might consider using old sheets on your bed or at least a set that you are not concerned about the oil staining.

You will want to have towels nearby and wear skimpy swimsuits. If swimsuits are not an option, you can use undergarments. Again use ones you are not worried about the baby/massage oil staining.

Where to perform:

You will probably want to perform this somewhere private. After all, you will be nearly naked as your perform it. Make sure it is a location that has good lighting. Your bedroom is typically a good choice, but may not allow enough room. The more privacy you have the less you will have to worry about interruptions.

How to perform:

Decide on an exercise that both of you will enjoy. It doesn't have to be the same exercise. If one of you likes weightlifting and the other likes aerobics, then do them (at the same time, but separately). The point is to get a good workout in before the sexy part of this challenge.

Once you have finished with your workout you might want to take turns showering or if you think sweat is sexy then just proceed. Slip into your "bodybuilder's attire". In other words, put on your swimsuit or undergarments. Don't be shy. The more you do this challenge the better and better you will feel about how your body looks. You might even have to go out and purchase smaller swimwear.

The next step is to oil each other up like the bodybuilders. Take turns covering each other in the oil you purchased. Cover every inch of each other's bodies with the oil. Make your partner glisten. The application of the oil is actually foreplay – so take your time and enjoy it. Move your hands sensually over your partner's body as you apply the oil especially when you are near erogenous zones. After you have finished your bodybuilder foreplay, which hopefully turned you both on, it is time for the show. Of course, your slickened bodies will offer wonderful sensations later, too.

Take turns flexing your muscles for each other. Don't worry about how you look. Just have fun with it. Make sure to appreciate your partner with applause or offering ooh's and ah's as he/she struts his/her stuff. If you are comfortable, strip down naked at this point and start flexing areas that normally are not shown during bodybuilding competitions ;-) For example, turn around and flex your naked butt cheeks for your partner. Laughter is okay as long as you are both having fun.

Mmmm, now it is time for the two of you as a couple to do some posing together. Let your bodies glide over each other as you flex and touch each other. Slide against your partner's thighs or enjoy the slippery back of your partner as you run your chest along it. You can add more oil at any time if you feel it has lost its slickness. Continue couple posing moving this activity into the bed – this is a great time to start adding kisses into the mix. Slide around each other like never before as you approach a more intimate show. Let all the parts of your bodies slip and slide around caressing your partner with your hands, arms, stomachs, genitals, etc. Slip into places you have never been - places like the back of the knees or armpits or wherever you both like. As you slip into making love try to keep flexing from time to time. Tense up your butt cheeks as your partner pulls you close or tighten your biceps as your partner holds on to them. Ladies remember to do those kegel flexes, too. Bring in any other items you would like to use during your play. **A note of caution – it is not suggested that you use baby oil as a lubrication for intercourse. It may make you prone to infection. If you want to end this challenge with intercourse, use a water-based massage oil that is safe internally.

During and after your intimate play, please be careful. Your bodies are slick and could be hazardous as you slide over each other or as you walk across bare floors or step into the shower. Ending up in the emergency room with doctors and nurses raising their eyebrows at your "bodybuilder" appearance is probably not on your agenda.

Lastly, think about how much better shape you will be in the more often you do this challenge. You can also prepare yourself a little better by exercising more often. Hey, what if you do this challenge as a way to gauge your success with working out and changing your eating? You could take measurements or weigh-in (remember muscle weighs more than fat – so it is possible to gain weight too). Make a pact with your partner to do this once a month or once every three months. See, feel, and relish your amazing changes.

More Than Finger Painting

Art has been around for a long time – perhaps, forever. It has been an outlet for sexual expression. The work the artist put on the canvass or carved out of the rock represented his/her passion. He/she created love in the world for many people to enjoy. If you have had the pleasure of creating a work of art you were proud of, then you know this feeling. In this challenge, you will take turns becoming a great artist.

You will put your passion and love into a visual expression for others to enjoy. During this time of creation you will become close and intimate with each other like you have never been before. You will see how each stroke of the paintbrush is important as well as each strike of the hammer against the chisel. You will become the artist, the tools and the canvass of expression. The two of you will become a living part of the art. Your passion will be on display from that point on and not just in art form, but in the passion between the two of you.

Items needed:

A drop cloth will be important to have to prevent paint getting on the floor or other things you do not want it on. You can find plastic ones at any local discount or hardware store.

You will need body paint. It is extremely important to make certain the paints you use are safe for your skin and washable. The washable paints should come off easily in the shower.

Canvasses are another item you will need. You can usually pick these up in bundles fairly inexpensively. Having a few extras on hand might be a good idea because they could rip or tear during the activities that will follow. Plus once you get started you might want to do more than one work of art or you might want to make a series.

You may also want to pick up some condoms or plastic wrap to cover areas of the body you do not want to get paint on or in.

Where to perform:

You will need to perform this challenge in a location that you can cover up easily with your drop cloth. You will also need plenty of room to move. Privacy will likely be high on your list. Your bedroom is almost always a great place to experience one of these adventures. Feel free to venture into other rooms of your home. Having a well-lit area will add to your experience though as you will probably want to see your artwork.

How to Perform:

Spread the drop cloth over the area you will be using. Get all of your paints and supplies ready and within reach. Remember to have your canvas near too. Make sure you will not need to leave the covered area until you are finished.

Both you and your partner should remove all your clothing. It might be more comfortable if you ensure that the room temperature is not too cool or too warm. If there are areas of your body that you are uncomfortable getting paint on, now is the time to cover them. If you don't want paint on your face, simply avoid it – but don't cover the mouth or nose either! After all, breathing seems to be pretty important to all of us.

Now, comes the fun part. Spread paint all over each other's body. You don't have to make it smooth. You can leave globs in certain areas; make it thicker or thinner here or there. Make sure to cover the genitals with paint and all the erogenous zones. (Remember those condoms or plastic wrap – you may want to have your genitals protected.) This not only will make your masterpiece great, but it also feels good. Once you are both covered with paint take the canvass and press it against one partner's body. Make an impression of his/her body on the canvass. Do the same with the second partner. Match up your impressions on the canvass so it is as though you are making love on the canvass. If you would like to make the painting less obvious rub the canvass around on your body a little, and allow this smearing technique to give your painting an opportunity to take on a new life. You can do this over and over again, if you like, using different colors to make your painting extra interesting.

Another option you might like is to put the paints directly on the canvass and then the two of you make love on top of the canvass letting the paint be directed by your lovemaking. Rolling around and moving to different positions can create interesting smudges in the painting. You could also use your partner's body as a paintbrush. You can use any and all parts from fingers to toes and from penis to breasts. Have fun with your passionate creation.

Once you have finished with your work of art you need to make sure to sign the painting as any artist would. Then, one last thing – give your masterpiece a name. You could create a bold and naughty name like "Our Fucking Masterpiece", or you could go for a softer name like "Colors of Passion". It is your artwork, your masterpiece; you have the right to name it what you wish.

De-Flower Me

The mention of the word "de-flower" immediately makes you think of a sexual situation. It is usually associated with a loss of innocence in our country. Yet, in other countries and cultures it is considered a right of passage from youth to adulthood. More than likely those of you reading this have already had your first sexual experience. So this de-flowering will be different.

This de-flowering will take a more naturalistic approach to the de-flowering. It actually involves flowers in the process. You will be using the powerful aroma and the relaxing qualities of these beautiful parts of nature to create a more relaxed state. Before starting, it would be beneficial to converse with your partner about any allergies he/she might have with flowers. It would not be enjoyable to have a bad reaction to the flowers or experience uncontrollable sneezing preventing you from enjoying this wonderful time.

Back in the sixties, groups that were referred to as hippies knew the power that flowers possessed. Many people still know this power, however, the majority of people just feel flowers are beautiful for the eyes to see and the nose to smell. After experiencing this scenario you will never look at flowers in the same way again. These beautiful treasures from nature will now become a link to great and amazing intimacy.

What you will need:

You will need as many flower petals as you can find – real flower petals. The fake ones will not give you the full power of this experience. You may have enough in your yard, but if not, you can venture down to your local florist and pick them up. Tell the florist you just need flower petals, and they can help you out.

A bottle of lube or your favorite massage oil is also needed. You might even match up the scent of the lube or oil with the flower petals you will be using. This will make the effect even more amazing. Nothing else is required, as you will not want anything coming between the two of you.

Where to perform:

Do this in a place where you can be naked together for a long period of time. The bedroom, as always, is a great place, but any place in the house will do as long as the privacy is there. Make sure the sheets or blankets you use underneath you are okay if the oil stains them. There is no need to ruin your good sheets. The color from the flower petals might bleed into the sheets or blankets also. So, this is another reason not to use your best linen.

How to perform:

Decide who will go first as the enjoyer of the flowers. You might even have a glass of wine to make a toast to each other and this experience. The first participant will then strip down completely naked lying in the desired location. It might even be more comfortable if you both become naked at this point. Have your partner lie down and relax as he/she prepares to be fused with the power of the flowers. The giver is to start by covering his/her partner's body with the flower petals you picked up earlier. Don't be sparing with these gifts of nature. Cover as much of your partner as you can. Stand over the top of him/her and let the petals rain down on upon the skin.

Once the petals are covering as much of the body as possible it is your job to remove each and every petal. The catch is you cannot use your hands or feet. You can pick them up with your mouth or use your breath to blow them off. The slower you can remove the petals the more excitement you will create for the later festivities. Save the erogenous areas and genitals for last and watch how your partner reacts as you remove the soft petals from these delicate areas. If you have trouble getting the petals to stay upon your partner's body, lightly cover your partner with massage oil first. This will make the removal process a little more difficult, but that might be even more fun.

Now that all the petals are removed it is time for you to massage your partner. As a bonus, put the flower petals in your hands and massage them into your partner's body. Take your time and let your partner enjoy the wonderful smell of the flowers as the power of these petals is introduced to your partner's skin. Again make sure you hit all the erogenous areas and the genitals with this power of the flower. Use this time to tease your lover into a frenzy. This will be rewarded back to you when you get your chance at absorbing the flower power.

Once both partners get to experience this wonderful journey into the power of flowers you may continue with your lovemaking. Throw some flower petals between the two of you as you become one. Breath in the smell of your lover combined with the wonderful scent of the flowers.

A great way to introduce this challenge to your partner and create a lasting memory is to use a ceiling fan. This works great and is a totally amazing thing to witness. Start by loading the blades of your ceiling fan with the flower petals. Put as many on each blade of the ceiling fan as you can for a more dramatic effect. Then invite your beloved to stand under the fan and await a surprise. Once he/she is under the fan, jump over and turn the fan on. Watch the amazing vision of your partner being rained upon by the beautiful flower petals. For best results make sure the fan is set to push the air up in the house. This makes the flower petal shower last a little bit longer. This isn't a memory that either one of you will forget for a long time.

Find My Nookie

What is "nookie"? Well, nookie is a slang word for having sex, making love, or just getting it on. Although this definition fits well within *Sexy Challenges* it is not the correct "nookie" I am talking about.

The nookie you are going to try to find is an amazing product by a unique company called Nookies Pleasure Apparel. You can find this company on the web at http://nookiespleasuresox.com. They have a wonderful assortment of sexy and enticing products. However, these sexy products are not just made for their visual appeal or their luxurious softness. They are scientifically designed to improve your intimacy. Below is a little more about Nookies Pleasure Sox.

Nookies, The Original Pleasure Sox bring women increased sexual pleasure with luxuriously sexy, naturally soft and scientifically temperature regulating sock styles for the bedroom. Nookies flirtatiously states the return of the good old-fashioned romp in the sack … only now with a 30% increase of a 'knock your socks off' orgasm!

Dutch scientists at the University of Groningen made a ground breaking discovery … women could increase their sexual pleasure simply by keeping their feet warm while making love.

That's great news except for one thing... socks are not created for sexual pleasure. Warm socks can be bulky and sweaty. Fashionable socks don't offer satisfying warmth. Now women can have temperature-regulating warmth in soft, sexy feminine silhouettes created specifically for more pleasure and satisfaction!

We combined the scientific research with indulgent quality to create an exceptionally unique product with a purpose... Nookies, The Original Pleasure Sox.

Women can slip into an experience with 4 distinct style personalities to match their moods and unleash their essence... Captivatingly Glamorous, Playfully Seductive, Confidently Suggestive and Innocently Flirty

Nookies Pleasure Sox ... fit beautifully ... are knit with our exclusive blend of fine natural and naughty yarns for endless wearability ... packaged with giftable boutique styles and original Pleasure Map for more enjoyment ... and are scientifically temperature-regulating for increased pleasure in the bedroom and beyond.

Just as "size matters", we at Nookies Pleasure Apparel feel "socks matter" too!

Nookies Pleasure Apparel combines over 40 years of experience in the sock industry with present day research to give women sexy sock styles in luxury, temperature-regulating yarns for increased sexual pleasure.

It is our commitment to create beautiful, elegant apparel that brings women more pleasure and fun.

Where to perform:

This can be performed in a multitude of areas. Obviously, the intimacy that will be the end result needs to be in a safe comfortable place for the two of you. However, the other part of this challenge might take you anywhere. It could be different rooms in your house, it could be at work, it could be in the car - the sky is the limit. The only restriction would be that the place you take action is safe from someone else disrupting the progression of this challenge.

What you will need:

The main ingredient is a wonderful pairs of socks from Nookies Pleasure Sox. Sure, you could use a cheap imitation, but believe me once you have a pair of Nookies Pleasure Sox the others will seem like you are wearing a sweaty old pair of gym socks. The only other thing you might need is paper and pen to leave your partner a note explaining this challenge to him/her. If you don't already have a pair of Nookies, then order a pair today at http://nookiespleasuresox.com.

How to Complete:

This is actually a game of hide and seek with a wonderful reward at the end. Once you have obtained your pair of Nookies, you need to divide the pair up. You take one sock and give the other one to your partner. You can explain the next part face-to-face to your partner or for a little more secrecy you can write it out on a note for your lover. Take the Nookie that you kept and hide it out-of-sight of your partner. The other one you will present to your partner with a stipulation similar to the following: "Once you find the mate to my Nookie, you will receive the best nookie of your life."

Now the hunt is on. Watch as your partner starts to tear up the house looking for the missing mate to your pair of Nookies. Make sure you hide the matching one in a good place because the longer it takes to find the mate the more excitement and anticipation you will have created. As mentioned above, this doesn't need to be done at home. You could present your lover with this challenge (and the mate) at work, in his/her car, or at any other location that is safe for the singular Nookie sock.

You can make the search really interesting by adding clues to lead your partner through various places. These clues could lead your partner straight to the sock or take him/her on a journey to another clue. The choice is up to you. One thing you might need to be prepared for is how long it takes to find the hidden sock. If you hide it really well, it might be days before your partner finds it. Make sure if you want the activities that follow to happen on a certain day, that you are prepared to lead your partner more clearly to the prize. For example, using the "you're getting hotter/you're getting colder" method you may have learned as a child when searching for a hidden object with friends is one option that you may choose to employ. Once your partner finds the hidden mate be sure the pleasure increasing sox actually get worn before the other aspects of your play begin. You don't want to miss out on the experience of increased sexual pleasure by keeping her tootsies warm.

No matter how you choose to play this sensuous game of hide-and-seek with your nookies you build anticipation within you and your partner for a fabulous session of lovemaking. Enjoy!

*A huge thank you goes to our friends at Nookies Pleasure Apparel for allowing us to write a Sexy Challenge based on Nookies, and for also making a high quality product that mixes physical intimacy and science.

Having a Ball With Sex

This will test your physical abilities as well as your ability to balance. Juggling a relationship is not an easy task and throwing a sexual relationship into the mix makes it much more challenging. However, I am going to take you out of your comfort zone and place you in a position to have fun and experience your intimacy in a whole new way.

Have you ever thought about how important exercise is to your relationship as well as your physical health? Well, this challenge is going to combine your exercise with your intimate activities for the evening.

After this, the term "exercise" will have a whole new meaning for you. You will also realize how important balance is to everything – not only in your relationship and life, but in your exercise and intimacy as well. After enjoying this intimate exercise and seeing how important balance is, you might start looking into yoga or other forms of exercises that combine your physical and mental strengths. Well, if you're ready, it is time to Pump You UP!!!!

What you will need:

You are going to need an exercise ball. If you don't have one, you will need to purchase one. Get one that fits your personal size and the size of your partner. If you are both short in stature, don't get the largest ball you can find. On the other hand, if you are both very tall, you might need to get the largest exercise ball. Take into consideration the weight that will be supported by the ball. Most exercise balls have a weight limit on the box; make sure your combined weight won't burst your bubble (or your ball in this case). You will also need a way to air up your exercise ball – after all, they do not blow up easily like a balloon. Most will come with a hand pump of some kind or if you have an air compressor at home that works too.

Other items you will need include lubrication and towels. Lube will help with transitions from position to position. While towels are for general cleanup and to remove any excess lube that might make the exercise ball a little slippery. Any other normal items you use during sex such as birth control or toys are also suggested.

Where to perform:

You want to have plenty of room to work on this challenge. Yet, you have to have privacy. Finding the right mix might be a little more challenging for the two of you. You will also need to find a place where you can move furniture out of the way to make sure you are safe. Obviously, you are going to be naked or close to being naked. So, you can't really do it in the middle of the living room if you have other people or children in your house. You might consider using a carpeted room in case you slip off of the ball – carpeted floors will make it safer for you.

How to complete:

What you are going to do is use the exercise ball to help you achieve a wide variety of new and exciting sexual experiences. The roundness of the exercise ball will allow you to get into many different positions that your bed will not allow. Using the exercise ball will give you a lot of different options and will also add a little more bounce to your lovemaking. The bounce of the ball will give thrusting a very different feel as the two of you use the spring for added excitement. A good example of this would be to use just a normal sitting position in which one partner sits on top of the other partner. Normally, one partner would be thrusting while the other one remains stationary or is lifting up and down. Adding the bounce of the ball to this thrusting will give both partners a sensation you might not have ever experienced. Besides the simple bounce of the ball you can also rock and roll a little.

Explore many different positions with the ball. Roll over and use a rear entry position, use your arms and legs to balance. You could even pick up a Kama Sutra position book and try out some that might not even seem possible in a bed. You can try different positions with the ball itself. You can roll the ball against the bed to give a little more stability or you can try to connect with the ball between your two bodies for some interesting challenges. You can use the ball to get into different positions for oral and anal sex also. Whatever you do, have fun with it.

A few words of warning here - always test your positions before you begin any vigorous actions to make sure it is safe. A trip to the emergency room is not on the top of anyone's list. Take it slow at first. You might get a check-up from your doctor before you take on this sexy challenge because the action of balancing takes a lot of strength and flexibility. Having a ball with sex can be exhausting, but in a really fun way.

Another option you might consider is to use the ball for foreplay. You could even bring different size balls into the mix to use on your partner's skin or just to add into different positions. Smaller balls could be used to give a massage to your partner before or after making love. The rolling action of a ball can be very therapeutic to the body. Whatever way you decide to do, *have a ball* with sex; just be safe and roll with it!

Amazing Orgasms

It is time to test your dexterity. You are going to get the most amazing ejaculation of your life. During ejaculation in men the contractions of the muscles and the ejaculation itself draws the testicle closer to the body. This is the natural reaction of the body. Finding a way to keep the testicles from being drawn up is going to be your challenge. While you don't want to mess around with nature, you would like to stretch out this feeling just a little bit longer. With women it is a little different, and all women seem to react differently so you might have to take some time and experiment a little. Both partners get a turn to be the giver and receiver in this challenge. If you are a same sex couple, then just take the areas that focus on your gender and take turns performing them on each other. Pushing each other past the point of pleasure will be an enjoyment for the both of you.

Where to perform:

You need to find a place that is private and comfortable. The bedroom is always a good place to start. However, feel free to branch out a little and enjoy the rest of the house or anywhere you feel comfortable. You might want to try a standing position for the males involved to allow them a different perspective. Women could also try a standing position, but I feel it might be a little easier for them to lie down and enjoy the sensations. Make sure the one administering the pleasure has a comfortable place to help bring amazing orgasms to you. Lastly, you will want a place that is stain resistant for any fluids that might be spilled upon the area. If need be, you can always throw down a blanket or towel to make all areas secure.

What you will need:

The first and most important thing you will need is a good lube. I suggest Sex Butter as it is a natural and wonderful product that is safe for you and it is safe to ingest - incase you want to perform this challenge orally. Without lube or with a poor lube you can end up chaffing and that can ruin the mood quickly. Sex toys can be beneficial as well as heighten the sensation in both males and females. You might want to invest in a cock ring for the man. It can help achieve the desired effect. Gather a few pillows to prop up against. This will help make both partners comfortable. You might want to have a towel or two handy, as you may want something to clean up with after the fun pushes the pleasure envelope. Your hands are the last things you will need, and are often considered one of the best sex toys ever - depending on how you use them.

How to complete:

Start by getting all your items needed close to your area of enjoyment. Let the first partner lie down, stand, or assume any position he/she feels comfortable in. If there is anything you are concerned about being ruined or stained, be sure to place towels over this. Place the pillows around in a manner to make you both as comfortable as possible while allowing you access to pleasure spots on your partner. If you want to restrain your partner, this is the time to do it. If you or your partner is uncomfortable with restraints, then you can just hang on to something like the edges of the bed or a towel rack. This will keep your hands from stopping the action. However, if you are going to use restraints make sure to have a "safe word". If you say the safe word, your partner will stop immediately! Make sure your chosen safe word is unique, but easily recognizable. If your partner has to stop and ask if you said the safe word, the mood is going to either be lost or at least severely interrupted. So, don't use words you might cry out normally when your pleasure increases. Use a word that has no relationship to sexual activity. You might use words like "bananas" or "silly putty".

A female partner should lie back while the other partner begins massaging her genitals. Slowly and softly massage her in the beginning, until you see that she is becoming aroused. As she becomes more aroused your

50

actions can become firmer and quicker. Focus on the areas she enjoys - the clitoris is a hot button for most women, but not in all women. At this point, you can introduce toys such as vibrators or dildos to the fun. You can use them on the outside of your partner or inside depending on what she enjoys. While the vagina is a great place to focus your attention, don't forget the anus and all those wonderful nerve endings down there that promote pleasure. You can begin to stimulate them orally if that is what your partner likes. What you do is not important. The reaction of pleasure is the most important part. Once your partner starts to near orgasm, have her grip the bed or anything near if she is not restrained. You need to hold on as well, and not stop until she can't take anymore or until she says the safe word. Some women might ejaculate and the amount can vary so be prepared for this just in case.

For a male partner you might want to use restraints depending on his strength compared to yours. Again, if you are uncomfortable with restraints give him something to grip onto, much like the bar on a roller coaster. Once he is ready to proceed, you can start stimulating him to gain an erection if he doesn't have one already. At this time you can apply a cock ring or a restraint to hold the testicles down to give him an amazing orgasm. Once the penis has achieved an erection use your lube to slicken it. If you want to use an oral technique, saliva is a great lubricant. Again, the product

Sex Butter would work for either method – oral stimulation or hand stimulation. Continue stroking your partner's penis in whatever manner you choose. You can also use toys at this point too. Don't be afraid to experiment with the anus. Most men will find this extremely erotic, but you should agree on this prior to experimentation. In most cases, the penis will begin to swell even more as it gets closer to ejaculation and you don't want to stop at this point. If you aren't using a device, such as a cock ring, to hold his testicles down, then you need to do this with your hand. Take a hand that is not stroking the penis and use it to hold onto the scrotum and hold the testicles from moving closer to the body. An easy way to do this is to make a circle with your thumb and index finger and wrap it around the area where the scrotum meets up with the shaft of the penis. Hold down on it gently as your partner begins to ejaculate. Continue these actions until your partner ejaculates and either moves away or yells the safe word in pleasure.

Once you both have experienced these amazing orgasms you will most likely want to revisit them from time to time to see how far you can push each other into the pleasure zone. Other things you might consider adding to this mix are using a mirror so your partner can watch the pleasure he/she is receiving. Lightly biting or spanking your partner can also heighten the sensation for some people. You can also use some of these techniques while your partner masturbates.   Using toys, holding down the testicles or stimulating the anus during masturbation will most likely increase your partner's pleasure.   Remember that your partner will be very sensitive after being pushed past the normal point of pleasure.   So, be careful when touching these erogenous areas.   Remember this is supposed to be a pleasurable activity.   Listen for the safe word and stop if you hear your partner say it.   With that simple rule you both will be able to reach new heights in your lovemaking.

Time Change

If you live in a part of the country where you have to change your clocks twice a year, you know how disrupting it can be. Just when you get used to the daylight savings time it is time to change those clocks again. There is supposed to be a reason for it, but I have not seen it yet. The only thing I see that it does is it makes the summer night seem to last forever.

Now, disrupting a pattern can be pretty annoying and bothersome. However, when we put that disruption into our intimate life it can add some excitement and needed change to our relationship. As we grow accustomed to our partner we tend to fall into a routine. Part of this is because we start to know his/her likes and dislikes and part of it is because we find time when things are most convenient.

This challenge will deal with getting you out of those routines and putting a little spontaneity back into your love life. Should your sex always be planned out? Do you feel like you have a window of opportunity where if you're going to get busy it has to fit in that time frame? Maybe you have kids and when they are in bed soon becomes the only time for adult playtime.

All these situations can be changed with a little effort and creative thinking. Think back to a time when the two of you just had to make love. You always found a time and place. Your passion was the driving force. So, where is that passion today? Are you afraid to let it come out and play again? Well, if you follow the challenge below you will soon see that passion return in a dramatic fashion.

Where to perform:

This challenge will call for you to make time for intimacy at different times of the day. You could be in your bedroom or the living room it doesn't matter. When the mood hits you don't worry about where you are. If you have the opportunity, make love in every room of the house. Heck, if you're a little more adventurous, you can move outside – just remember to seek privacy.

What you will need:

Basically, for this challenge all you need is what you normally use for sexual activity. If you use birth control such as condoms, then make sure to have some with you. Lube is another wonderful thing to have on hand when it starts to get hot and heavy. You can even strategically place sex toys around to have them readily available when the mood hits. With this challenge you might need to plan a little ahead, but I would love to see you be ready at the drop of hat.

How to complete:

The main focus of this challenge is to break out of your routine and switch up your sex life a little. Most couples get in the habit of having sex at the same time of day. On average that time is right before bed, which makes sense, as you are both together at that time and usually wearing a lesser amount of clothing. However, having sex at the same time can become monotonous and unfortunately, can begin to feel like a chore to some people. While sometimes this is brought on by necessity, due to children or work schedules, there are still ways around it.

For starters, the simplest way to change up the time you make love is to set the alarm for an hour earlier than you normally get up. Morning sex can really start your day off right. You hear of many people getting up early to exercise, well sex is a form of exercise. You can take turns waking each other up with kisses and caresses. Just be careful. Sometimes people can get jumpy and even grumpy when you wake them up unexpectedly. Take the time to slowly arouse each other for your morning session of intimacy. Think about it, if it is passionate and wonderful, you are going to carry it around with you all day.

Another great way to mix up the time a little is to use your lunch hour to make love. This can be a really anticipated event if the two of you talk about it beforehand. Agree to meet at home at a time that works for both of you with the knowledge that sex is the main course at this lunch. You will be surprised at how excited you will become on the drive home. Imagine how quickly the two of you can rip each other's clothes off as you find the perfect place to make love. This lunchtime sex is good too because for a good part of the year your kids will be at school during the daytime hours. This gives you free reign of the house for your sexy lunch.

You can also find more interesting ways to change the time you make love. Take turns setting the alarm for the middle of the night to wake up and make love and then fall back asleep. You can also make plans to send the kids to the movies with friends or grandparents. This can give you a good couple of hours to make love in the early part of the evening. If you like hot sweaty sex, you can take a break from lawn work to make love before returning to the mower. You can even get really creative and pick a random time out of a hat and then find a way to make it happen. Don't be afraid to use personal time from work to have sex, after all that is very personal and worth the time off.

No matter what way you find to change the time of your sexual adventures, you will find that it improves the overall process. Putting effort into your intimacy is a relationship builder and it will also make you appreciate the next time you don't have to worry so much about it. Use all your resources, like babysitters, time off, insomnia, etc. to take this challenge and soon you will be rocking around the clock.

Hippie Beads

Oh the sixties and their free love movement. If you are not familiar with the hippies from that time period, you should do some studying on them. They were radical in their thinking of love and peace over war and destruction. Doesn't it seem amazing that love and peace was considered "radical thinking"? Shouldn't it be a given that love and peace should rule our world? However, the hippies had to find wonderful and interesting ways to prove their point. So many great things came out of the sixties. We turned away from having to follow the norm and broke out of the molds that our society was trying to get us all to fit into.

One of these wonderful concepts that came out of the sixties was a positive mindset about sex and intimacy. Even though we have a long way to go we are now free to choose our sexual orientation, free to explore our sexuality in ways we never have. In this challenge, you want to focus on something that the hippies didn't invent, but they expanded our minds and our sexual experiences.

Hippies loved to wear their beads making fabulous necklaces out of them. They would use amazing shapes and colors to express their individuality. Now, these wonderful necklaces were not the only reason that hippies enjoyed beads. They introduced or perhaps, reintroduced our culture to using beads as a pleasure instrument. Not only can you create and give a wonderful massage with a string full of beads, but you can become more intimate with the beads and your lover.

I doubt this was the sole purpose for the hippies' beads, but you have to admit it must have been handy to have them around their necks when these intimate situations would arise. Instead of having to find them in the drawer beside the bed, they were right there. This might not have been the main explosion of the sexual revolution, but perhaps, it had a hand in bringing toys into the bedroom.

Go find your Jimi Hendrix or Doors' songs and get prepared to take a blast back to the past and experience a little hippie fun.

What you will need:

You will need some beads. These are not the ones you find at your local store. I am talking about beads used for sexual pleasure. Check out any online adult toy store and you will find several different varieties, colors and shapes of these little beauties. They have beads for massaging, vaginal pleasure, and anal pleasure. Pick out some that you and your partner are comfortable with and order them. Other ways I suggest you set a sixties' mood include black lights or colored lights, your favorite music from that era, incense and maybe even some tie-dye. The sixties, in my opinion, created some of the best music ever and you can find it on iTunes as well as other places. Make sure you remember the lube though - those beads don't lubricate themselves.

Lastly, some words of warning: Make sure the material your beads are made of are safe for your body. Make sure that they are properly constructed for the areas you will be using them. You don't want a trip to the emergency room. That could be expensive, uncomfortable and embarrassing.

Where to perform:

Your home is a great place to perform this challenge, but I suggest getting out of the bedroom when you can. You could even create a love den if you have a spare room to enjoy. Of course, you can venture out to your living or family room. Just make sure you have your privacy. You might want to have plenty of room in case you want to dance together naked or roll all over the place letting the passion consume the two of you.

How to complete:

Once you have your beads with you then you can set your time machine back to the sixties. I know most of you don't have a time machine. So, you will just have to imagine. Consider having a little wine to help loosen things up a bit. However, do not drink too much. Your intimate play won't be as enjoyable if you pass out or if become nauseated. Turn your music on so that it loops or plays continuously. Set your mood lighting. If you aren't using black or colored lights, then turn your normal lights down low or use candles (or flameless candles).

Get your groove on by dancing around to the music. Let yourselves explore each other's bodies. Let the music consume you and feel it move through your body and your partner's body. Relax. Know that pleasure is coming and welcome it with not only your body, but with your mind. Once you feel alive and invigorated by the music and the passion it is time to experience the beads. You will take turns, but let one lover go first. Use the beads to massage his/her body rolling them across large areas like the back, chest, and legs. Move to the erogenous areas and let the beads caress and tantalize. Make sure you have the proper lubrication within reach and begin beading your partner with pleasure.

For a male partner you can wrap the beads around the shaft of his penis letting them roll and bring even more blood flowing to the area. Play with the beads and his testicles at the same time rolling them together in your hands. If you and your partner have agreed to do so, reach over and get your lube and gently slide the first bead into his anus. If this is his first time experiencing this it might be a little difficult to get him to relax. If so, try putting some lube on his penis and stroking him as you try again. Once he is receptive of the beads, you can begin to move more inside him. At this point you could bring him to climax for an amazing sensation and you can do this with your hand or orally. Once he has experienced all he can take then slowly start to withdraw the beads. Be careful not to rush and allow him to experience the pleasure of each bead as it exits his body.

For a female partner this bead sensation can be doubled. You can use the beads in both the anus and vagina (however not the same set, do not move bead from the anus to the vagina, as the bacteria from the anus could cause infection in the vagina). The beauty of this is you can insert all these wonderful beads into your female partner and then still perform oral sex on her. Always listen to your partner's moans or words as you insert beads into her. She may be able to handle all the beads you have or she may only enjoy a small amount of them inside. You have to communicate to know for sure. Bring your female partner to climax either with your hand or orally and let her enjoy the sensation of the beads as she orgasms. If she offers you guidance or a hand make sure to follow or allow her to proceed. The pleasure you are aiming for is hers. Once she is finished with her orgasm just like in the male partner remove the beads slowly and gently. Allow her also to enjoy the pleasure of the removal of the beads. This might even create another orgasm or two during the removal.

Once you both have had a turn you might want to make love or just relax and enjoy the euphoria that the pleasure has brought about. Either way is fine. Let the music roll and listen as you gaze into each other's eyes or into the night sky. Hopefully, after this experience the words "hippie" and "beads" will bring shivers to your body like never before. Just take your time and enjoy them each and every time. One thing hippies did teach us is that our pleasure is worth every second we put into it and that it is our right to enjoy what we were supposed to enjoy.

Lastly, I want to give one more warning. Never put anything inside your vagina or anus that isn't made to do so. Make sure the items have the proper safety, such as a flared bottom, to make sure they are easily removed. Use lots of lubrication on anything being inserted into the anus as it does not create it's own lubrication, like the vagina. GO SLOW! The end result is much better when you take your time and make sure everything is safe and comfortable for the both of you. It never hurts to check with your doctor if you have questions or to make sure you are healthy enough for sexual relations.

Frozen Panties / Underwear

This challenge is based on an old slumber party ritual that most of you might have participated in during your youth. The person that fell asleep first at our slumber parties had this unwanted event happen to them. However, in the version we are sharing this event will be more of a turn on than a turn off.

Sometimes ice can be used as an extreme way to get each other excited. The differences in hot and cold can drastically increase blood flow to the areas that sensation is focused upon. When those areas are around erogenous zones or genitals it can bring a person to arousal very quickly. I caution everyone that does this challenge to stay within reason. While frostbite isn't a real concern, I don't want you exposed to the cold for too long either.

Once you start this challenge it is unlikely that you will have to worry about anyone falling asleep any time soon. In fact, with any luck this experience will have you up for a good part of the night.

Where to perform:

Probably the best place to do this is at your home. Most of the reason for this is you need privacy and a freezer. Another reason to perform this at home is that it will take a little while for the freezer to work it's magic. So make sure you plan ahead.

What you will need:

You will need a pair of panties/underwear for each of you. Next you will need access to water. You can use tap water or bottled water. It is a good idea to get a couple of balloons or balls to help keep the underwear in shape. A spray bottle would also be helpful to test the amount of water you need to use on your undergarments.

How to compete:

As you might have guessed by now you are going to take turns freezing each other's panties/underwear. You will see who can endure the cold on their private parts the longest. Start out by selecting the underwear the two of you are going to use. Use your spray bottle to dampen both pair. If you feel really brave, you can completely soak both pair in the sink. Wring out the excess water before placing them in the freezer. Use blown up balloons to place inside the underwear to help the underwear keep the shape of your body. The balloons will start to loose air in the freezer so if you have a ball the correct size, it might even work better.

If you are sensitive to the cold and not sure how much you can handle, try just placing the underwear in the freezer without making them damp first. This way you don't get a total freeze-out when you put them on later. After dampening the underwear, place the balloons or balls inside them and place them in the freezer. Leave both pair in the freezer for at least a couple of hours or longer if you have planned ahead. When you remove them they should be stiff and frozen, but the fabric should still give a little. This will allow you to slip them on. Frosty will take on a whole new meaning for you.

If you like, time each other to see who can keep the frozen underwear on the longest. You can make a small intimate wager on the outcome to make things a bit more interesting. Add pleasure by quickly enjoying some form of intimacy right after removing the cold items. See how quickly you can warm your partner up. Oral sex can take on a new life after this event. Your hot breath can quickly warm those frozen body parts. This can also be an interesting sensation for your mouth and tongue.

If the idea of freezing your underwear is too farfetched for you, start out by taking a towel and tearing it into strips. Put the strips through the same process as above and place them on different areas of the body to get the desired effects. Other variations could be to switch back and forth from hot to cold underwear. Put one pair in the freezer and the other in the dryer and then take turns going from one extreme to the other. Just as you feel the chill of the frozen panties remove them and put on the steaming hot ones from the dryer. You will be amazed at the changes as you body adjusts to accommodate these extremes. (Be cautious of too hot or too cold!)

As with all your sexy challenges make sure to take your time and error on the side of safety. Don't push the edge too far and stop if the sensation gets to be too much. Make sure you are healthy enough for sex and if there is any question check with your doctor.

Sacrifice To The Gods of Passion

Many of us worship something in our lives be it a God or something else. Yet, how many of us dedicate our lovemaking to that God or the Divine? For centuries, various cultures and indigenous people have offered a sacrificial virgin to their gods. These sacrifices were designed to keep the gods from being angry. Why they used a virgin, I am not for sure, but it probably had something to do with purity and innocence. Maybe it would have been better to give the gods someone with a little more experience?

In this day and age, we are not going to offer up a life, but we can offer up an orgasm. This orgasm will be different from the normal ones achieved during sex or masturbation. Your partner will become your God or your source of the Divine and you will honor him/her/them by giving your body and your orgasm as an act of worship. You might just experience a deeper more powerful orgasm than you ever have before. The God(s) of sex and intimacy is rarely worshiped in this manner. So, they will most likely be filled with pure joy as you offer and experience a powerful orgasm.

The most important part of this challenge is to make sure that what you are doing feels good for both you and your partner. Any sex or intimacy "God" that you might worship has the goal of pleasure in mind. So, make sure that pleasure is at the forefront of your desires.

If you do not have a God or idol that you worship, you can make one up or go to the library and find one to give your orgasm to. You might even consider worshiping the God/Goddess inside of each of you as the recipient of the pleasure. While this sexy challenge might seem a bit odd, very similar practices have happened for years from couples making love in the fields to promote a good crop to passionate lovemaking as a protective measure before entering into battle. If you look back in history, you will see that using orgasm as a means of prayer has been around for a long time. I am just bringing it back into the light. It seems we have gotten away from it due to the censorship from religion.

This challenge just might help you achieve an out-of-body orgasm or you might achieve a closer and more intimate relationship with your partner. Either way it will be amazing.

Where to perform:

I suggest you use a room in your home in which you can safely be fully naked and not be interrupted. You will also need a good deal of room to stretch out. More often than not couples make love in their bed. Try to find someplace different even though your bed is probably quite comfortable. By making love in other areas you bring your sexual energy into the rest of your home.

What you will need:

Lubrication is a must for this challenge. Select a kind that does not dissipate quickly. Towels for clean up are always a good idea too. You might consider candles, flameless candles, or some kind of mood lighting. Soft lighting is wonderful and you get to see your partner as the two of you turn your orgasm into a sacrifice.

How to complete:

Choose who will go first in this ritual. You can flip a coin or draw straws, but whatever the outcome know that the other partner will have his/her chance, too. The first chosen is the first to offer an orgasm as a sacrifice. To sacrifice your orgasm to the sex or intimacy God(s) you must find a way to orgasm using parts of your partner's body. You can use his/her arms, legs, butt cheeks, cleavage, thighs, or any part that works for you. The only rule is there is to be no penetration or self-stimulation with hands. Once you find the body part you wish to use in your sacrificial ritual you can proceed to lubricate it and your genital area. Start moving your genitals slowly over the lubricated part of your partner until you become aroused and excited. The partner going next should remain as calm and relaxed as possible as the sacrificial participant manipulates his/her genitals. Don't offer assistance. Only offer the services of your body and the willingness to help with this sacrifice. Once your partner has achieved orgasm offer a towel for clean up, then switch roles.

You might have a little trouble trying to think of places on your partner that you can orgasm without any assistance. Some of the obvious ones are the penis in cleavage, penis in butt crack, or clitoris rubbing on thigh or forearm. Break free of the normal and try something totally different. Rubbing your clitoris on your partner's nose or the tailbone can stimulate you to orgasm quite nicely. You can use the joints of you partner if you're a male such as where the elbow bends or the back of the knee. Challenging areas for both sexes could be using the feet and toes to bring about orgasm. Watch and feel the sensation as your partner gives you the gift - spreading love all over you. Take turns and get all you can out of this venture and soon the sex or intimacy Gods will be calling for you to orgasm while you are part of one another. Don't be discouraged if something doesn't work for you. Just move to another area and try again. Soon you will find a spot that calls to you.

You can also honor the God/Goddess in both of you while you do your normal lovemaking. Simply set the intention before you begin. Go all out. Use candles, incense, or body paints to decorate your room and each other. Chant, sing or howl if you feel like it. Let the feeling inside you come out and enjoy the connection you will make with the God/Goddess.

Sexual Golf

Golf is one of today's most popular games. Millions of dollars are spent on golf courses every year. Not only is it popular, but it still carries a lot of prestige around it. Many view it as a wealthy person's sport and not for the lower class. Thank goodness with new programs this is becoming a thing of the past. I, however, am not focused on improving the game or making it more accessible to the masses. My focus is incorporating the aspects of this great game into your intimacy. I want you to find a way to enjoy your sexual passion in a similar manner as the many golf enthusiasts out there today. Heck, it might even help some of you get your partners to leave the course a little earlier so you can play a round at home.

Sexual golf will help the two of you enjoy an extended week of sexual excitement. You will be playing nine holes of this kind of golf over the next nine days. So rest up and take plenty of vitamins. You are going to need them.

This challenge will put a little sport into your lovemaking. Both partners will be choosing and scoring the selected activities for each evening. The partners will take turns making up the courses and how they will be performed with the ninth course being given to the winner of the first eight courses. The focus will be on trying different positions while avoiding activities never before tried. For example, if you don't normally have anal sex, don't put it into one of your courses. You will be cramming a lot of sex into the next nine days, and you don't want either partner being sore for the next course.

Where to perfrom:

Contrary to the title you will not be actually playing golf. You will use your home as the course or any other location you have the space and feel safe. As with the designing of any great golf course you will be looking for areas around your house to use as part of the course. Items that you normally might not have thought about using during sexual intimacy will become props or "hazards" in your new game.

What you will need:

You might want to look over a sexual positions book to get some new ideas. These books give lots of insight and even directions in how to get into the position. Once again as with all the challenges lubrication is something you will need to have readily available. With the amount of times you are going to be intimate over the next few days you very likely will need it. If one of you truly needs a day off, consider it a "rain out" and return to the game when you are back up to par. If you are lucky enough to have a golf course nearby, you can go in a pick up a couple of their score cards. You are going to use these to keep tally of your sexual golf experience. If not, you can print some off the Internet or make your own. Heck, you can even just use a notepad of any sorts. You will also need a notepad to right down the number and procedure for each hole of your course. You can even copy or print visuals of sexual positions to help get your point across to your lover. Lastly, (this is totally optional) you can get a trophy for the winner of your sexual golf tournament.

How to complete:

Each partner gets to plan out four holes (sexual activities). Each hole on the course is a different sexual activity, position, or event. Remember not to include things your partner and you do not normally take part in. If you haven't had oral sex, you can avoid it, unless it is something you both want to try. However, you don't want to just put down oral sex as one of your "holes". Make it a little different. Maybe you have oral sex in a chair or while one of you is leaning over the couch. This is where you need to be creative. Maybe you want to try to have sex on a piece of exercise equipment or see how long it takes you both to melt a few ice cubes while making love or see how much you like sweaty sex by turning up the heat in your bedroom. Each of you gets to plan out four super sexy and creative "holes" (sexual activities). There should be a variety. The more different they are from each other – the more exciting they will be.

After each partner has planned out his/her four holes with specifics details, you need to find a way to choose whose to start with. You can flip a coin, roll a die, or run a race as long as there is a clear-cut winner. The person that wins gets to put his/her holes as numbers 1,3,5,7. The other partner will number his/her holes as 2,4,6,8. Now you both make up a special hole. This is something you want to especially enjoy. You won't show this hole (activity) to your partner. Instead, each of you will seal up your special hole (activity) in an envelope with your name on the front. These will be for the ninth hole and will be decided by the winning score.

Both partners look over the first hole's specifics and get ready to begin play. Warm up if you need to and take a few practice swings, but not too many - you don't want the hole over before you even start. Perform the activity as specified and then take a few moments after the passion to give the activity a score. You will score the activity - not the performance of your partner. You both score each activity. The score reflects whether you enjoyed the sexual activity or not.

If it is your hole you score it between one and five with one being great and five being lousy. If it is not your hole, you score it between one and three. One being great and three meaning you didn't enjoy it very much. Put the scores on the scorecard and then put it away. Continue with this process until you have completed the eight holes presented before the two of you. A word of caution here - please be totally honest with your scoring. Don't try to weigh the scoring in your favor. You both win in the end - so don't cheat.

Tally up the scores after the last day and see who has the lowest score. Just like in real golf the person with the lowest score is the winner. He/she hasn't won yet however. You still have the last hole to go. This hole will decide the winner of your sexual golf tournament. Take the envelope of the person with the lowest score at the end of the eighth hole and open it up for the ninth hole activity. Once the envelope is open it is set in stone and the last hole is ready for play.

Perform the hole just like the others and score it in the same way as before. Once you score this last hole you can tally up the totals to find the lowest score and the winner. Present the award (if you have one) to the winner and then treat yourselves both to a great evening out.

The secret of this sexy challenge is to be completely honest and to be happy if your partner wins. After all this is a win-win situation because both of you will get to enjoy the moments and activities together. You might even pick up some new exciting things to begin using on a more regular basis. No matter how you look at it sexual golf will get you trying something new and exciting, and that is never a bad thing in a relationship.

Oh, one more thing - remember not to wear your golf shoes to bed. That might be a little dangerous.

Breast Cancer Awareness

Sexy ways to guard against breast and testicular cancer in honor of National Breast Cancer Awareness Month

Cancer has robbed so many people of life. There is not one type of cancer that is worse than any other; they are all difficult. However, there are a couple that stick out in the area of sex that we can help screen for in our normal sexual activities. Breast and testicular cancer are both types of cancer that you can have a fighting chance against if you detect them early. That is why I am dedicating this sexy challenge to detecting and surviving these two cancers. Yes, I know there are several other types of cancer that affect our sexy lives such as prostate cancer and ovarian cancer. While these two, also, greatly affect our sexual health they are not as easy to check for by the normal person. Obviously, all cancers can affect our lives, but these two have some tried and true methods of checks that can not only be exciting, but should be at least part of your foreplay once a month.

I am not making light of these checks. Instead, I am hoping to get more people to do them on a consistent basis and if they happen to get excited performing them, that is a bonus.

In this challenge I am going to give you several ways to enjoy your turn at checking your partner more often. The playful checking will lead to a good amount of fun afterwards. However, if you do find a lump don't freak out, go ahead and enjoy yourselves, but as soon as possible get your partner to get checked out. Error on the side of safety and remember this is my attempt to help detect breast and testicular cancer early.

Where to perfrom:

This challenge should be performed in your home - in your bedroom with just the two of you and some soft candlelight. Some other variations might have you jumping in the shower together or finding fun positions to check your partner. The important part is to be some place that feels safe for the two of you.

What you will need:

It might help to use lube, lotion, or massage oil. Allow your hands to slide across the breasts or testicles. Get some warm towels to wrap your lover in once all the exploration is over. You might even turn up the heat a little if it is cold where you are.

How to complete:

If your partner is female, you will check her breasts for any lumps or spots that might not feel normal in her breasts. The first suggestion is to get your beautiful woman into a nice hot shower. Let the water run over her body tracing all her curves and creases. Once she is totally wet begin soaping her down using lots of soap coating her breasts. Gently start caressing her breasts slowly at first then applying a little more pressure. Let your hands cup and feel each wonderful breast as if you were feeling it for the first time. Enjoy, but make sure to do a good check. Take the tips of your fingers and gently, but firmly press into the breast tissue. Cover the entire breast including around the nipple and under the arm. Once you have adequately checked each breast proceed to enjoy other areas of her body. Then make wonderful love to her.

Your second option is to get the lube out and get things a little slick. First gently, but firmly, press your fingertips against her breast tissue as above. After you have checked each breast pour a generous amount of lube or massage oil over each of her breasts. Warming the lube first is a wonderfully delicious idea. Let your hands glide over the breast with complete coverage making sure to go slowly to feel and enjoy the massage for both of you. Again, if you find any lumps or anything that doesn't feel right, don't freak out. Continue with your massage. After you finish making love check the area out. Rub each breast with small circular strokes from time to time. Spend a good amount of time doing this because it is also foreplay. Run your open palms over the nipples and find interesting ways for your partner to experience different kinds of touches to this erogenous zone. If your partner starts to arch her back, it might be time to massage other areas of her body. Again, try to do this exercise in foreplay at least once a month. If you do that, you will be prepared to notice anything as soon as it arises. Below I share an illustration on how to perform a breast exam for you to study.

If your partner is a male, the foreplay is similar. First of all, you will be checking for lumps or masses again, but this time on the testicles. The first option again is to hop in a hot shower and soap up your man. The testicles are very sensitive and checking them might be a little uncomfortable to your man. Go slow and take your time. The testicles should move away from the body with the hot water. This gives you an excellent opportunity to check them as they dangle in the scrotum. Gently roll them around between your fingers getting the feel of their egg shape. I suggest seeing if you can get an erection out of your man to give you more access to the testicles. Let the testicles rest in your hands and move from one to the next. Explore them and get to know them. This will be a huge turn on for your male partner so be prepared either to quickly move him to the bed or to offer a hand job in the shower.

The second option to check again requires a good amount of lube. I reiterate that the testicles are sensitive and gentle action is required as you roll each delicate testicle between your fingers. I also suggest again stroking the shaft to get the penis out of the way by achieving an erection in your male partner. Once you have given your mate a wonderful and thorough check take advantage of the erection you have created and get a little pleasure out of it yourself. If that is not in your plan, then consider a hand job. It is a wonderful alternative and you have the lube very handy if you decide to go this route.

Just as with the breast exam/foreplay exercise it is a good idea to do this on monthly basis. If I can help one person detect these types of cancers early enough to help them, I will be very happy. Sex is very important in our lives, but our all around health is vital. Blending your exams with foreplay will make it more likely that you will complete the exams.

This is a beautiful way to show love for your partner. Now during your intimate and passionate time together you can also be focusing on each other's health.

Getting Intimate with a "Ghost"

It is a simple fact that the paranormal fascinates many people in this world. We look for things to scare us or make us uneasy. We want the excitement of fear, and yet, we want to know that it is all okay. Getting our adrenaline pumping is the same action we look for from sex. However, we don't want our sexual experience to scare us. We want the blood pumping in all the right places. How can we combine the two elements and have a wonderful time together?

Role-play is such an interesting part of physical intimacy. There are thousands of costumes out there that can turn on just about anyone. Sexy witches, gladiators, horny little devils just to name a few that could get the sexual juices flowing. Most of us have a favorite that would turn us on. Halloween time makes it easier as there are so many costumes available. Tons of people dress up for Halloween, but what if it isn't Halloween? You can still pull those costumes out or create new ones to use in your intimate play.

This challenge is aimed at trying to get you to feel like you're being intimate with a ghost. No, you are not going to pull out the Ouija board or go to a graveyard at the stroke of midnight, but you are going to get a sensation that will leave you wondering.

Where to perform:

This challenge needs to be performed in a place where you can lie down. A bedroom or couch in your living room will work fine. It also needs to be in a place where you can light some candles. I prefer you use flameless candles for safety purposes. Candlelight really helps set the mood for this experience.

What you will need:

The first thing you need for this challenge is a sheet. Be sure it is a sheet you are not worried about ruining. A plain white one is a great idea because it gives a better effect, as you will see later. Plus, sheets with puppies or flowers all over them will lessen the experience. I suggest a bottle of your favorite lube and a towel or two for clean up as well. (Optional) A recording of spooky noises like doors creaking, wind howling, moaning etc. can add to the mood. That is if you are looking for a spookier feeling.

How to complete:

Have your partner lie down. Take the sheet and drape it over your partner covering his/her entire body. Make sure to cover his/her head too. It is very important to do this. It helps with the illusion. (Caution: Make sure your partner can breathe comfortably under the sheet!)

Turn the lights off and light your candles or turn the candles on. If you don't have candles, you might consider the lowest lighting you can achieve in the area. If you decided to go for the sound effects, now is the time to put the recording on and let the music/sounds help shift the mood. Instruct your partner to lie perfectly still and let the spirit take control. Start by breathing on him/her through the sheet focusing on his/her normal erotic zones. Areas such as the ears, mouth and neck work great. You want to give that goose bump feeling as he/she feels your warm breath coming through the sheet.

Start to rub him/her lightly through the sheet. Slowly and lightly touch the body so that it is almost as if you were not touching your partner at all. See if the body starts to react. Watch the sheet to see if your male partner starts to get an erection. Either sex might start to show excitement by the nipples becoming erect and visible through the sheet. Keep this up for several minutes tantalizing the senses and allowing the excitement to build.

Once your partner starts yearning for more, touch him/her. You can start letting the ghost in you have its way with him/her. Start to fondle the genitals and breasts enough to let your partner know that you mean business. Don't put your hands under the sheet though. Keep the sheet between you at all times. If your partner is male, start stroking his penis through the sheet pulling hard on it. If your partner is female, start finding the lips of her labia and playing with them through the sheet. You can start using your mouth to stimulate the nipples still keeping the sheet between them and you. You can even move down to the genitals and continue with oral sex while stimulating through the sheet. Once you get him/her really excited it is time to bring him/her to orgasm. If you need your lube, quickly slide your lube under the sheet and generously coat the genitals. Then return to the outside of the sheet. Stroke the penis or massage the clitoris through the sheet.

You can still use your mouth if you like giving oral sex through the sheet and if you are really into it, try to have sex with the sheet between you. A really thin sheet might help you achieve this goal. Yet, be careful not to chafe your partner. The important thing is to make sure you bring him/her to orgasm. Watch the sheet as it soaks up the love juice. You may very well have been able to orgasm too. If you don't at first, take the opportunity to do so while your partner is still covered. You will both be satisfied and then you can spend the rest of the night talking about your ghost story. Of course, you could switch positions so that you may orgasm or you can try it another night so that you experience what it is like to be intimate with a "ghost."

In Specially Marked Packages

This challenge is a great way to introduce new and exciting things into your sex life. How many times have you wanted to try something new only you have been too scared or nervous about asking? I have heard this all too often that once something new such as a toy is introduced into the relationship both partners get as much enjoyment out of it as the other. This leaves them wondering why they didn't get the courage up to suggest this long ago.

I understand that this task can be a little nerve racking. Any time you suggest a new way of stimulating your partner you face the fear of rejection. That is where this challenge comes in so handy. I offer you the opportunity to introduce this new toy in a funny and non-threatening way. This challenge will give your partner the chance to understand your interest in a specific toy outside the context of your bedroom.

In this way, not only will you get to present him/her with your ideas, but you can also present this idea when you are not even around. With a little planning and the element of surprise you can let your suggestion fall right into your partner's lap. Once you perform this challenge there will be no way your partner will not know what toy you want to try in the bedroom.

Where to perform:

This should probably be completed inside your home. Most likely it will take place at your kitchen table or wherever you eat your breakfast. You could also do this in a public restaurant, however, you better be sure your partner is the type that is easygoing or you may upset him/her greatly. Also, if you have children or other people in your home, you will need to be highly discreet.

What you will need:

You will need a box of your partner's favorite breakfast cereal. This needs to be the kind that only he/she eats. The bigger the box the better because the area inside needs to allow room for your item. You will need a plastic sealable bag. Make sure you get a large enough size to handle the prize. Lastly, you need to have a sex toy or item that you want to introduce into your intimate relationship. That could be a vibrator, a specific lube, a masturbation sleeve or anything that strikes your fancy.

How to complete:

This challenge may be one of the easiest I have ever put together to complete. The reason being is because it only takes one partner to set it up. You can set up the challenge and it might happen that day or it could be a couple of weeks before you get the results. It all depends on how much cereal your partner eats.

After selecting an item/adult toy you would like to try, drop it into the plastic bag and place it in inside the box of cereal. Be sure to include a note inside the bag with the item. You can say something like, "Look Honey! You won a prize! Let's use it." or "Honey, I would love to try this sometime." Whatever you want to say it should let your partner know you are interested in using the item.

When placing the plastic bag inside the cereal box be careful. You will need to initially remove some cereal so that you may place the item towards the bottom of the box. Yet, you do not want it to be obvious that the box has been tampered with. Be sure you put the cereal back in the box on top of the item. Covering it just as the toy surprises in a children's cereal box would be. Place the box back on the shelf in its normal spot. Now sit back and wait.

Avoid trying to push the cereal on your partner. You want him/her to find it naturally on his/her own. The scenario can play out many different ways. You might be sitting at the table with him/her when the item falls into the cereal bowl or maybe you will be at work when it happens. I hope your partner will not only understand and get excited about the prize, but might get a laugh out of your presentation.

You can have some different variations of this challenge. If your partner doesn't eat cereal, you could pick a different type of food that comes in a box. Heck, you could even put it in the chip bag. You could also make a fake sticker that says "Special surprise in each box!" to put on the outside of the box. If you are unsure of what item to get or would like to know what he/she would like to introduce into your sex life, you could put a gift certificate in place of the item from one of the many safe and exciting sex toy shops. (There are a large number of them online now too.)

You could even package your item with other items such as tickets to a performance or sporting event. This might sweeten the deal even more. You could also try multiple toys or homemade coupons for pleasure-filled nights of passion. Use your imagination and bring the fun to your relationship.

This challenge adds a little humor to the nervousness of suggesting a new toy into your sex life. If the humor doesn't thrill you, think back to when you were a kid. There was always excitement about getting to the toy or prize in the box. When you got that toy out of the cereal box, you at least tried it once didn't you? So, have fun and add some sparks to your relationship.

Human Vibrators

Vibrators can be a wonderful experience for anyone. However, it might just be a wonderful experience for the both of you - at the same time. A good number of women nowadays use a vibrator either when they go solo or as an aid during sexual intimacy with a partner. The sensation and the hum of a vibrator can be very stimulating for some women. Constant stimulation of the clitoris with a vibrating device can help some women reach a magical orgasmic place.

Yet, even in this day and age of sexual information some partners are still scared of sex toys and feel that the vibrator is going to replace them. So, I ask you - How many vibrators can kiss softly on the neck or hold you tightly during climax? None. Understand that sex toys are just tools to build your sex life. You wouldn't build a house without a hammer would you? The use of tools is to help you not to replace you.

Vibrators are not just for the ladies either. Men you can enjoy the pleasurable feel too. This challenge will make you feel like a god/goddess, and it will help your partner feel like a warrior instead of a caddy for your sex toy golf bag. You might just have to fight your partner for control of the vibrator after it is all said and done. The sensation of sex is a wonderful thing and this is just another way to enhance it.

Where to perform:

This challenge needs to take place somewhere that you feel safe. You might not get it right the first time so you want to be able to take your time. Choose a place that will not allow interruptions. As always the bedroom is a great place to start this challenge. Of course, mood lighting can be beneficial as well so that you will be able to see what you are doing.

What you will need:

You will need small sized vibrators. Bullet vibes or even the new vibrating cock rings will work. The new vibrating cock rings are wonderful and inexpensive to throw away after use. You might want to have about 3 or 4 of these wonderful tools around and you will see why in a bit. You will need rubber bands or ponytail holders. Ponytail holders work better because they are softer. As always make sure you have lube on hand to help out if dryness is a problem.

How to complete:

What you are going to do in this challenge is turn your partner into a human vibrator. This will show him/her the advantages of stimulation during the use of a vibrator. The first thing you are going to do if your partner is a man is attach one of your vibrators to the base of his penis. Use some of your rubber bands or ponytail holders to wrap around both the penis and the vibrator - wrapping them together. Make sure not to restrict too much blood flow to the penis and avoid prolonged use of this tactic without a break now and then. Turn the vibrator on and let your man start to feel the sensation vibrating his penis. Take another vibrator and place it between the cheeks of your partner's behind. Get it as close to the anus as you can without any penetration. Fire up that vibrator and hope that your partner doesn't ejaculate before you get to enjoy the vibration also.

If your vibrator has a flared base you can penetrate the anus with it, but it MUST have a flared base. Make sure your partner is comfortable with this idea first though.

If your partner is a woman, instead of attaching a vibrator to the penis attach it to her fingers. Once you have all the motors humming away on the vibrators then it is your turn to play. Start using your partner's penis or fingers as your own personal vibrator. Running it over the areas you typically would with a normal vibrator. You will be amazed at how the skin acts at another form of stimulation as it vibrates upon your body parts.

Don't stop there. Feel free to have sex with the vibrators attached. This is truly a pleasure for both of you as it gives you a whole new sensation. And, don't forget about oral sex. Slide his vibrating penis into your mouth to give him an experience he won't soon forget.

You might also consider trying to share the vibrator. Try to keep it between the two of you using only your bodies (no hands), and see how talented the two of you are. Once comfortable, you can also have a sit and play session where you both sit on vibrators as you play with each other. No matter what or how you choose to play just be sure to enjoy your special time together.

Rolling the Dice

One of the biggest complaints people have about their sex lives is that it always takes place in the bedroom. The reason most people have sex in their bedroom is easy to understand. For starters it is safe, it is usually not a high traffic area or a place that people just barge into, it is comfortable, they have their normal bed, their comfy sheets and pillows to make their stay even softer, and they love making love in their bedroom because it is convenient. All of their toys and/or lube are in a drawer close by so that they can enjoy them quickly and easily.

As wonderful as the bedroom is, sometimes you need to break out of this mold to understand how truly wonderful it is. Getting out of your comfort zone will allow you to appreciate that feeling when you return. On the other hand, you can get a new rush of excitement from making love elsewhere. And, venturing out to other areas of the house offers opportunities for different positions. You may try chairs, tables, the couch, the tub, the shower, etc.

Start looking around your house today and I bet you can find someplace that might just turn you on a little as a lovemaking destination. So many people are afraid to try this, but it can add a great deal of excitement to your lovemaking.

If nothing else it will make that particular time memorable. Making love in your bedroom is great, but it blends in with all the other times. The time you make love in the chair is something the two of you can remember for many years to come.

Where to perform:

Well this is kind of up to chance, but most any room in your home is good. The whole idea is to make love in a different place. Therefore, if you still want to stay in the bedroom, you can try the floor or the edge of the bed or maybe a chair in the bedroom.

What you will need:

All you will need is a pair of dice. Not anything fancy - just the ones with the numbers one thru six on them. Remember to have things like your lube, toys, and condoms at your fingertips too. Oh, and you might want to find some blankets. You may want them for warmth or for a quick cover-up.

How to complete:

To complete this challenge you start by assigning each area in your house a number from two to twelve. (If you want to stay in the bedroom, simply make adjustments and assign parts of the bed, parts of the bedroom, etc.) Below is a sample list:

#2 - In the Living Room

#3 - Sitting in the Office Chair

#4 - On the Kitchen Table

#5 - In the Shower

#6 - On the Porch Swing

#7 - In the Recliner

#8 - Against the Refrigerator

#9 - In the Closet

#10 - In the Car

#11 - In the Front Hallway

#12 - On the furry carpet in the Family Room

Once you have your list completed then you can pretty much guess what happens. You roll your dice and see what number comes up. Then presto, that is where you are going to make love. No questions, no backing out. The only thing you have to do is find the ideal time that you can be naked and frisky in that area of the house. This challenge can go on and on. After you have made love in one of the locations, you can replace it with a new location or choose to keep it on the list if you both enjoyed it.

Other variations could be that you assign a sexual position to try to each of the numbers. You could also assign sexual favors to each number to get straight to the action. However, that seems pretty similar to some of the novelty dice already on the market. Of course, you can use this little method to get you away from the dreaded, "What do you want to do tonight?" Use the dice to pick what you have for dinner or what movie you are going to rent this week. You could even use this method to sort out the chores for the week – who does the laundry, dishes, grocery shopping, etc. Just have fun with this challenge and add something new to your relationship.

Sexual Meditation

Meditation is a great way to get in touch with your inner self. Within the silence and stillness you can discover lots of things about your true being. You can release the demons from your past and become one with the energy of the Universe. While most meditation is designed to be an individual practice there are several ways to incorporate your partner into this state of bliss. Tantric practices have the lover's breath where you breathe in the essence of your partner as you meditate and circulate your breathing between the two of you. Massage is another way couples can take turns meditating while the other partner stimulates and releases pains that are physical. However, most couples' meditations stop at the point.

This challenge will push past that area of just being as one in spirit and will combine it with a sexy twist. Time and patience are important here, as you must demonstrate self-control to get the full experience. Part of the sexiness of this challenge is to feel and enjoy sensations as if they were foreplay. Once you understand the pure joy of this slow and passionate challenge you will come back to it over and over again.

As you journey into this challenge, understand that the intimacy of your sex life will only be heightened by this practice. Letting yourself explore the touch and letting your partner share in that space between the physical and spiritual will create a special connection. Sexy meditation might release past feelings of pain or joy so accept the wonder associated with it and simply bear witness to unexpected emotions. Focus on being one with your partner. Go into this challenge with your mind open and accepting.

Where to perform:

Do this in a warm and comfortable place for the both of you. It needs to be a place where you will not be interrupted and can feel safe being naked with each other. I suggest the bedroom because of the ability to control the environment. You can set the heat or coolness of the room as well as the lighting. The bedroom is also a sacred place for most couples, a place where the two of you retire to be alone. The bedroom is also great because it holds a sexual essence and sexual energy from past experiences with each other. The Zen of the bedroom helps bring a special touch to this challenge.

What you will need:

While nothing here is required you can enhance the mood with a few items. Candles (natural or flameless) allow you to see your partner in his/her natural state. They create soft and precious flickers of light, which caress both of you. Please always be careful with candles!

Lube is another great tool for any sexual experience. This challenge is slow and will not create a high rate of friction, but the lube might help the beginning of touching in some areas. Plus, the lube might come in handy after the meditation when the friction might get a little more heated. Massage oil might be desired at the beginning depending on how much focus you put into the massage section of this challenge. Soft sheets and soft towels are a great touch and are even more special when they touch your body. Soft and mellow music can help reduce outside noise, and incense can offer a beautiful aroma to the space. While you want the comfort of your bedroom you still want to make it feel like a different place. Use as many of these means as needed to achieve that feeling.

How to complete:

Make sure the room temperature is comfortable – neither too hot nor too cold. Remove all clothing. Once you are both naked meet in the center of the bed without getting under the covers. Spend a few minutes together in this space with your eyes closed. Get close to each other without touching letting your auras or energies blend together outside of your bodies. The touching will come later. See if you can sense your partner's body, breath, and energy as you quietly sit together. Try to synchronize your breathing and relax your body within this state. Let your mind think of nothing except the breath and the space inside your body. Take as long as you like during this relaxation and flowing part of the meditation. Once you are both calm and relaxed you can move on to the next part of this challenge and enjoy the sensual aspects of massage during meditation.

Decide which one of you will get massaged first. That person should lie on his/her stomach to start. Begin the massage by applying massage oil if you have it and start working it into the shoulders and neck area. Use deep pressure or a lighter pressure – whichever your partner prefers. Move to the lower back and the arms taking time with each area and making sure to massage both arms and all areas of the back. Pass over the rear end and do the same on the legs and feet. Move up the legs slowly and work on the rear end.

Once you have hit all areas on the back turn your partner over and start on the front. Again focus at the start on the arms and legs. Move gently to the breast and chest area and carefully start massaging the breasts of your woman or pecks of your man. At this point, avoid the nipples as you will come back to that during your sexy meditation. Next, move down to the genitals and use light stroking actions to stimulate to the point of arousal. No penetrating women or stroking the shaft of your man. Just use light caresses to send the tingles into the area and increase the blood flow. Once the first partner has completed his/her turn it is time to trade and the opposite partner does the same exact steps to get the first partner ready for the events to follow.

Once the massage or warm up is done it is time to begin the sexy meditation. Meet again in the center of the bed and intertwine your legs so that your genitals are touching. In a male-female relationship, put the head of his penis touching the entrance of the woman's vagina. Male-male relationship will have both penises touching each other and in female-female relationship you will have to get really close to get the outer lips of the labia to contact each other. Once the connection of touch is accomplished stare deeply into one another's eyes. Breathe deeply and synchronize your breath. Breathe in each other's breath and focus on the areas touching each other. Start to close your eyes and continue breathing and focusing on the touching parts of your body. For about five to ten minutes, continue this breath work on becoming one in your relationship. Once out of this first area you will start to work on the erogenous zones and start speaking the words of sexy meditation to your partners.

Pick out a few phrases that you can whisper to your partner as you allow him/her to meditate on your love and passion. Things like, "Your pleasure is my desire," "I enjoy being one with you," or "You are so sexy to me." You can use others as long as they are positive and spoken softly. Once you have your phrases down you will start stimulating your partner's erogenous zones as he/she meditates and you speak your soft words. You will have to know your partner's erogenous zones so you might have to do a little research before this challenge. However, I hope most of you know them by now. Areas such as the nipples, genitals, neck, anus, and lips seem to be very common ones. Of course, some out of the way places might do the trick. Places like the armpits, back of the knees, toes and palms are often quite sensitive. Whichever ones he/she needs, try to hit as many of them as you can.

Once you have covered the areas you want it is time to move on to the areas that will test your meditation focus. Start with the nipples. Put your genitals upon or between her/his nipples and speak to your partner as he/she focuses on blending your penis/vagina into him/her. Move to the anus and either place a finger at the opening of the anus or your penis. Let your partner breathe in your sexual essence as you speak. Remember do not stimulate the anus at this point. Just place your body part there and allow the heat of it to be felt. Move to either the vagina or penis and melt your vagina/penis into your partner's. Make sure he/she is breathing and feeling the sexual energy climbing. Now reverse your positions and let your partner meditate on your phrases and touches as he/she reaches into sexual meditation. It is normal for you to become sexually aroused during this process. So don't worry as your penis swells with excitement or your vagina begins to get wet and juicy - this is part of the process.

Once you both have been giver and receiver it is time to combine all that sexual meditation into each other. Let your emotions free and devour each other. Let your sexual essence spill all over each other. Dive into oral, anal, or whatever kind of sex you enjoy. Feel the passion between the two of you as you have most likely reached a special place for both of you. Feel how different your touch seems. Enjoy the special extra caresses you give each other and melt into each other with reckless abandon. The space you occupy is shared with your lover now and the passion should be even deeper than before.

You have now had and enjoyed a sexual meditation. Hopefully, this will not be your last experience with this and you will soon start making it a regular practice between the two of you or should I say you should make it a regular practice for the oneness of your relationship.

Making Love Uphill

We have all heard that trying out different positions can increase our sexual pleasure. Just the thought of trying to find different and exciting ways to be able to perform sexual intercourse is fun in its own right. Not only can you try different positions, but you can use items like pillows and wedges to get you and your partner into different angles for penetration. Then you can even venture out of the bed and try having sex standing up, in the shower, or bent over a chair in the living room. These are all great and wonderfully exciting things to try.

However, this variation on the changing of positions is a little more involved than just getting into a new position. This challenge will take a little work, but will be worth it in the long run. You are going to think outside the box a little and yet stay in your bed. This will have you feeling and experiencing your intimacy in a whole different way. Not only will you have a couple of different options, but you can start adding the items mentioned in the paragraph above to help out too.

Pushing a boulder up a hill is not much fun – just ask Sisyphus (brush up on your Greek mythology to find why this king had to push a boulder up a hill for eternity). But, how hard can making love up a hill be? Sound interesting? Well, get prepared. With a little work you will soon have you and your partner not only up the hill, but gasping for breath as you are having an orgasm.

Where to perform:

This challenge should be performed in your bed. You could use the couch or another bed in your house, too. Even one of those blow-up mattresses could work. Pick an area that you will feel comfortable making love in.

What you will need:

You will need some pieces of wood that you can cut into one-foot squares or several hard cover books that meet those dimensions. The reason you need the pieces of wood or books to be this size is because you need them to be stable and support a couple hundred pounds of weight. Make sure you have enough pieces so that when they are stacked on top of each other you get at least six inches of height. You will need two sets of wood both equal in height.

How to complete:

First get your pieces of wood set. You will need to cut them and connect them in some fashion to be stable. You could nail them together, glue them or even screw them together. Make sure you try to reach that six-inch mark for both sections of your wood.

Have your partner help and you will both enjoy the excitement of getting this challenge underway. Lift the head of your bed up so that the blocks of wood or books can be placed under both legs of the bed where your head rests. Your bed should now be slanted up and your head should be above your feet. When you start making love you will be making love uphill. See how differently it feels to be climbing up your partner as you engage him/her in intimacy.

If you feel that six inches isn't enough for the two of you, feel free to get some more pieces of wood or add some more books under the legs of the bed. Make it as challenging or interesting as you like. But, remember to keep it stable and use safety precautions. See how differently it feels as you thrust upwards instead of doing it on a level area.

You can also try doing it downhill by switching the way you are laying on the bed. It might give you quite a rush by having your head lower than you genitals during sex. Another option would be to just raise one side of the bed so that you create a different feeling altogether. If you have a smaller bed or are using a couch you might even be able to soar to further heights. You could raise these lighter pieces of furniture to much larger heights for incredible sensations. Always make sure to check for safety however. Double check your items before you begin and make sure they will hold up to the weight of the situation.

I do believe that all the options will create a different feeling as it will change the blood flow for both partners. Maybe you should just try all the ways to see which one is the best for the two of you. Don't be afraid to use straps to hold on to. Enjoy the difference in the position of your bed. This will also alter the angle of penetration so be prepared for a different sensation.

Become the Warrior

Most people have the fantasy of being a warrior or being swept away by a warrior. Maybe you want to be a warrior princess or just want to release the savage inside of you. Whatever it is that draws you to this image, it is primitive and basic. Being able to let go of today's social status and get into the feeling of being half naked and ferocious is liberating. Letting the true nature of your sexuality out in the most passionate way is wonderful.

Nothing is sexier than the warrior as he/she paints up his/her face and prepares for "battle." In this challenge, I want you to pretend it is the night before the battle and you are enjoying the passion a couple might have before the brave would leave. There is heightened passion because there is always the possibility that he/she might not come home. Let yourself unleash this passion that would be there if you did not know whether or not your brave warrior would return. Succumb to the feeling that it might be the last time the two of you make love. Let the passion rise to help your warrior in battle.

Your primitive animalistic nature will love this challenge. It will take you to another place and time. You can get caught up in the fantasy. Consider what effect drums might have upon you as you feel their rhythmic beat? Will you lose yourself in the arms of your lover as you stare deep into his/her eyes? Will you be transported back in time or to another life?

All of that depends on what you believe. However, this challenge will let you experience these feelings as you stroke the muscles of your brave warrior. Believe me when I tell you that this challenge might go off the chart for you. Grab your spears, shuck your shoes and get ready to experience loving your warrior.

Where to perform:

This challenge needs to be in a darkened room. Make it somewhere that music being played will not affect others in the house or the neighbors. You don't have to use the bed. You might throw some blankets on the floor to make a more realistic warrior living arrangement.

What you will need:

Get some body paint. I suggest basic white. The darker colors seem to be a little harder to get off of your skin and tend to stain sheets and the shower floor. Some baby oil can give the effect of a sweaty body. It will make your body glisten and become sexier in the dim light of your quarters. I, also, suggest flameless candles. They produce the same flicker as real candles and can be easily and safely placed anywhere for dramatic effect. Find some music with tribal beats - you can download them from iTunes or pick up a CD at your local store.

How to complete:

Start by deciding who will be the warrior. Then apply the baby oil to that person until he/she glistens all over. Turn the lights down or off and turn on the flameless candles. Once you have the candles placed around the area your sexual ritual will take place, turn on your music. Turn it up as loud as you can and start to feel the beat.

It is time for you to prepare your lover for battle by sharing your love. Apply the paint to your lover with your fingers. Stroking stripes across his/her cheeks and forehead. You can move to other areas of the body if you feel the desire. Once you have your warrior ready for battle step back and admire how sexy he/she looks. Let your partner paint you as well in a similar way if you want to.

Beads, necklaces, feathers, etc. can add more and more to this challenge. You can even find out special ways or symbols to paint on your lover. Take pictures of each other to remember your warrior night of lovemaking if you desire. Enjoy this as you are now ready for whatever battles you face.

It was often believed that making love to a warrior before battle would help protect him/her. The belief was that the energy and passion of love would guide the warrior to make the right choices and bring him/her back safely to the home. Are you going to take a chance of your warrior not coming back home? I would suspect not. Put all the passion you can into the lovemaking of this evening. I am sure most of you out there are not going into actual battles, but this can help in your day-to-day challenges and "battles" that we all face.

Does your partner have a big presentation to give the next morning? Maybe there is a situation that is a little unnerving your partner has to deal with. It might even just be dealing with traffic jams or difficult customers. These are all examples of modern day battles. So, if you think we don't have battles to prepare for in this day and age, you have overlooked some very common ones. Protect your partner and honor him/her as he/she goes off to battle. At least this way, your lover will go with a smile on his/her face and your love and passion in his/her heart.

Cleansing Ritual

Most people think of sex as a spontaneous thing that just happens. Your hormones get the best of you, and as if you were animals, you attack each other. This is not all bad when it happens, but most of the time in a relationship that doesn't happen. More often than not you have a target date for your sexual encounters. Maybe you even have a sex night or schedule sex into your lives when you have time. This is very popular nowadays as couples' schedules are busy and don't often allow for spontaneous sex.

However, it is important not to lose the fact that sex should be special in a relationship. It shouldn't become a chore or just something you need to do because it is on the calendar. It should still be exciting and fun. How do you balance having time for lovemaking and spontaneity? Is there a way to increase the appeal and excitement of sex?

What if I told you that taking your time and slowing down your sexual experiences can make them better than they have ever been – even if they occur on a scheduled day? You probably already know that foreplay is a wonderful and exciting thing that should last until both partners are ready for intercourse, but have you considered what happens before foreplay? Is there a warm-up to foreplay to help get both partners in the mood?

The focus of this challenge is to show you that treating yourself and your partner to a wonderful sexual experience starts before you slip into bed. Not only does it start with the rising of the sun, but as your intimate evening draws closer you can increase the romantic and sexy mood by doing what is called a cleansing ritual. This will allow you to enjoy each other free of any distractions, any negativity, any grit and grime from the day. You will feel fresh and ready for a wonderful night of lovemaking.

Where to perform:

This challenge will start in your bathroom and continue into your bedroom or any room you feel comfortable making love. The cleansing ritual can take many different directions, but they all lead to that wonderful vehicle that will take you to orgasmic bliss.

What you will need:

For this challenge you can go about it one of two ways. You can use the normal shampoo and soaps that you have at home and use on a daily basis or you can go out and purchase different shampoo and soaps that have a drastically different smell and feel to them to share with your partner. I recommend the second option. Get lotions to use to soften your skin and make sure you have a razor to shave any areas you want to shave. Remember the toothpaste and mouthwash too. Have a robe or something special to put on after your cleansing ritual and emerge from your royal bath feeling like the god/goddess you are.

How to complete:

This challenge needs to involve both of you. Take turns doing the cleansing ritual or do it together. After cleansing, one or both of you should go about setting up the room by turning down the sheets, laying out a blanket, lighting candles, turning on soft music, etc. Take your time doing the ritual. Rushing will take away from the experience.

Whether you take a shower or a bath, be sure to allow your body to relax in the magical water. Bathe yourself in the warmth of the cleansing, refreshing, rejuvenating water. If you like taking time to soap your body in a sensual way, do so or allow your partner to do it for you. Slowly, make sure to clean all parts of your body. Use a sponge, washcloth or your hands to make sure every inch of your skin is cleaned and refreshed for your partner. Take the time to wash your hair and make it smooth and soft for your lover to touch. Take time rinsing the soap and shampoo away from your body just as you took time to apply it.

Once you feel that you have cleansed yourself head-to-toe you need to find a large fluffy towel and dry yourself. Just pat your skin with the towel. Don't scrub your skin. If you purchased any lotion, now would be the time to smooth it over your skin. Rub it in thoroughly. Join your cleansed body with your partner's cleansed body and relish in what follows. Present your body to your partner in the most immaculate fashion - clean and prepared for pleasure, with the scents and feel of royalty. This new excitement will carry you to many different places as you kiss your way up and down the ultimate path to an amazing orgasm for both of you.

Checking the Undercarriage

Many people spend a lot of time figuring out different positions for sex. It can be fun and exciting to try new things in your lovemaking. It keeps things fresh. Why don't you put this into a different aspect of your love life? Some people will wear different clothes to get into role-playing to change things around. Others might look for different locations in the house.

Great ideas, but how often do you consider finding different positions for foreplay? Foreplay is such an important part of sexual intimacy. Yet, many fail to treat it as such. You can use your hands, mouths, toes, or any other body part to stimulate your partner. So why don't you use them all to your advantage?

In this challenge, you will discover a great way to enhance your foreplay. This interesting concept will bring about different sensations for both you and your partner. I encourage you to try this and then expand on it. Put in your own twists and turns to make it special for the two of you. With just a little change in your foreplay patterns you will bring excitement beyond belief to you and your partner.

Where to perform:

This challenge can be performed anywhere that the two of you participate in sexual activities. You can use it in the bedroom, on the couch, or on the living room floor, etc. Adding different places to this challenge makes it more of a special event. Yet, starting out in the normal place that you make love might be the best idea. Then after you get comfortable, you can branch out and move around your home.

What you will need:

For this challenge you will need whatever items that you normally use during foreplay. If you use lube, then use lube. If toys are part of your foreplay ritual, then break out the toys. I don't want to disrupt what works in your relationship. I just want to heighten the experience of your foreplay. This simple twist on your normal foreplay will bring a new awareness to your senses.

How to complete:

This challenge is simple and fun for both partners. You can start out clothed or naked - whichever you prefer. If you typically start your foreplay in your clothes or pajamas, then do that here also. If you start your foreplay naked, then start out naked. Get comfortable in your normal place of intimacy and then prepare for the twist.

One partner is going to use foreplay first on his/her partner. He/she should lie back on the bed. The receiver of the foreplay will hover over the top of the giving partner on all fours. This will allow the person performing the foreplay to enjoy the body of the person hovering above in a much different manner.

If your partner is male, then you will have his penis hanging above you. However, there is much more to focus on than just the penis in a male partner. The testicles and scrotum will be much different hanging above you. This will also allow easy access to the anus and buttocks of your male partner. Remember to also play with his nipples. They are sensitive too, and are quite often a great source of joy in males. This position for foreplay allows you to caress in many different ways with both hands. You can reach the back of the neck or stroke down the spinal column with ease.

Your male partner will be very appreciative for the focus on his body. You can also rotate around underneath your male partner to put special focus on certain areas. You could perform oral sex to the point of climax in this position. That will likely drive him wild. But, this position could also allow you to give him a different hand job as you either stay below him or venture up top to reach around and perform the hand job. No matter what you choose to do, it will be a different experience with him in this position.

Now, if your partner is female you can start out in the same way. Of course, you will obviously have some different body parts to play with. You can perform oral sex in this position to give her an extraordinary orgasm. Understand that this position gives you the opportunity to use both hands while stimulating your female partner. You will have an easy time reaching her anus for heightened stimulation if this is something you both enjoy. The breasts hang down and you can kiss and lick around the whole breast and chest area. This offers a very different feel of the breasts for both of you.

You will also be able to caress your female partner in many different ways such as caressing her back and rear end with both hands. Make sure to caress her legs and arms also. A light feathery touch can drive some women, as well as some men, wild with sensual pleasure. You can also position yourself differently to achieve different sensations for your lover. You can slide in sideways or crawl under her from between her legs. All these little angles and differences will give her a new and exciting experience.

Make sure to allow time for both partners to enjoy this exciting means of foreplay. If you do not get both of you in during one session of lovemaking, then make sure to allow the other partner his/her turn during your next intimate time together. The beauty of this challenge is that it puts a different twist into your normal intimacy without having you step too far out of the box. Throwing in this little extra way of foreplay into your lovemaking will quickly add some spice to your relationship.

Change in the Weather

Nothing is as unpredictable as the weather. One minute it can be sunny and warm and the next you are staring down the face of a tremendous thunderstorm. There are so many different types of weather that can affect our day-to-day life. We can have blizzards, tornados, hurricanes or a rash of other natural weather predicaments. Have you ever thought about using these weather conditions to improve your sex life?

Does the sight of lighting make you feel energized? What about the crack of thunder? What weather condition do you find sexy? Is it snuggling up during blizzard conditions in the dead of winter? How about the swoosh of the wind as it blows through the trees? Granted weather can be a bit scary at times, but it can also cause an adrenalin rush.

With this challenge you will soon find yourself excited to see that a snowstorm is moving in or that those clouds might bring a downpour. You will find a new reason to watch the weather forecast. With this challenge within your thoughts you will soon start getting excited by the changes in the weather. You might even start finding out how to do a rain dance.

Some people want to put as much spontaneity into their sex lives as they can. This challenge will help you do that. It will make each and every day a chance to perform wonderful spontaneous sex depending on how the wind blows. Give in to the weather forecast and start experiencing the true power of nature.

Where to perform:

This challenge works best when you are at home where you can watch the local weather forecast in comfort. It can also be done on vacation or any place where you can be alone and watch the change in the weather.

What you will need:

You will need some type of media for this challenge be it television, radio, or Internet. Of course, you may just happen to get caught out in a storm and be able to find a secluded spot. You will need anything else that you normally use during sexual intimacy. Things such as condoms, lube, and sex toys are a few examples of things to have on hand and ready for these weather changes.

How to complete:

This challenge is quite simple – just make love when the weather changes. Have a conversation about what elements of nature you find the sexiest. It could be a thunderstorm or a snowstorm. Find out what your partner likes! Then you make a pact together that every time that condition arises and you two are together you make love. Yes, this challenge is pretty simple, but it takes the control out of both of your hands and puts it in the hands of nature.

This is not the only time you have sex, of course, but these are added times to become physically intimate. You might just have made love and a couple of hours later whatever weather condition you have decided upon might come about. Well, you can't ignore your weather condition. So go back and make love again. As we all know, even though they might predict rain showers it doesn't mean that it is definitely going to happen.

A fun way to get more out of this challenge is to set certain activities for certain weather conditions. For example, you could both agree that if a thunderstorm comes up that you will have oral sex. Another option might be that if it starts snowing you have to make love by the fireplace. You can even make a competition out of it. Where at the first sight of lightning the partner who gets completely naked first gets to choose the position of your lovemaking for that evening.

Another fun way to use weather during intimacy is to let it guide your adventure. For example, during a thunderstorm you could decide that every time lightning fills your room, you change positions. During a big storm this could get quite interesting and exhilarating.

You can also use the results of a weather condition to guide your lovemaking. You could have set sexual activities to perform based on these results. Amount of rain or snow could be the deciding factors on what your intimacy will bring for that day. For example 1-2 inches of snow could equal sex in a hot shower, while 3-4 inches of snow would require a rousing session of cunnilingus. Any amount of snow 5 inches or above would require you have sex on the kitchen table.

This can be twisted into whatever you like and enjoy. However, you will still be at the mercy of the elements. Just hope that if you pick rain as your choice you don't have a drought. If that happens, you might just have to learn to do that rain dance after all. You should also check the area that you live in as to how often your chosen weather condition arises. Some of the top areas for rain have rain 160 plus times a year, while some of the driest only have about 30 to 40 days of rain a year. So choose wisely. Or choose a different location and keep an eye on their weather. Whatever works for the two of you the best is what you should do.

Sexy Shopping Spree

This is a wonderful way for the two of you to connect and learn about each other's sexual desires. I suggest that every couple do this at least once a year, if not more often, to keep their sex life fresh and interesting. This is a wonderful opportunity to share your sexual preferences and desires with your partner. Whether or not you are normally comfortable talking about these things this challenge offers you an exciting new activity to enjoy with your partner. Wait – you are too uncomfortable to talk about it? Well, guess what? You don't actually have to talk about it for this challenge. Take this opportunity to be more open and emotionally vulnerable with your partner in a different way. You can learn so much and deepen the bond between the two of you.

There are a vast number of places, many of which are online, where you can purchase sex toys and items of pleasure. That makes this challenge easier. Decide whether you would be more comfortable searching online or visiting a brick-and-mortar store. When shopping for adult toys some of you may be shy about browsing in an actual store. Yet, others of you may prefer to see the item up close and personal vs. only seeing it online. Virtual stores allow you to browse from the comfort of your home, but don't allow you to hold the item in your hands. Depending on the site, you may make mistakes when ordering an item. You need to pay close attention to the description before ordering. Of course, ordering online allows you a level of privacy that shopping in a physical location does not.

Whatever your taste or personal views this adventure is sure to ignite some great moments in your relationship. It will get your heart pumping in several different ways. Not only will it allow you to shower your partner with gratitude and love, but that gratitude and love will be reciprocated to you and your pleasure.

You can use this idea for birthdays, anniversaries, or any other special day. You will end up with huge smiles on your faces. You might find yourself waiting for the mail carrier or getting a special package of your own very soon.

What you will need:

You need to find a place that sells intimate items of pleasure. I suggest using an online presence, but if you have an actual store close to your home and you are comfortable going in to browse then you may choose that one. Once you find your desired store, the next thing you need to do is make sure they sell gift certificates. The gift certificate is an essential part of this challenge.

Where to perform:

If you have chosen a store online, you can complete this challenge without ever leaving your house. If you have chosen an actual store near your home, you will have to venture out at least once to this store. After the shopping, you will be able to complete the rest of this experience wherever you choose. Depending on the items purchased you can tailor the place to the item. For example, if you choose something to use that needs a bed then you may choose your bedroom as the location. Now if you choose something with a little more fantasy to it, you might want to venture out of the house and get a hotel. If you are really feeling wild you might even make love in your car. The choice is yours or your partner's.

How to complete:

The first thing you need to do is purchase a gift certificate or gift card from the chosen store. The amount of the certificate or card is up to you. Of course, more money will allow for a bigger selection of items.

Then, go out and purchase a normal greeting card that expresses your love for your partner. You can also make a card if you want to add a little more personal touch to the process. Inside the card, you will give your lover the instructions he/she needs. You can adjust the words, but here is a wonderful suggestion to put within your card.

134

Honey, please take this gift certificate and access this wonderful store. Use the money on the certificate to purchase items that YOU are interested in bringing into our intimate play. Do not ask me for help, this is YOUR Choice. I will be open and loving to whatever you choose. Do this in private, and do not tell me what you have purchased. The only catch to this is you have to have the items sent to ME! Yes, you have to put my name on the package so that it is delivered to me. Once I have received the items I will not speak of them until we have a chance to use them. I love you and I am excited to help quench your desires.

Now leave this card on his/her pillow or someplace he/she will get it when you are not around.

Once you get your package in the mail do not say a word to your partner. Survey the items inside and begin making plans for a fun filled evening for the two of you to experiment and enjoy. Make sure you have adequate time to use the items in the package or at least set up other times to use the items you don't get around to the first time. You might be surprised at the items your lover chooses to enjoy in your intimacy. It really is a great gift to the both of you. Who knows maybe you will be the recipient of the next gift certificate so you can express your most intimate desires.

Super Soak-Her or Him

As adults we very seldom get to act like kids again. We have strict guidelines at work, we have chores to do at home and we have to be role models for our children. If you are a person, who can act silly doing all these things, that is wonderful. However, most of us can't find that happy place that we used to experience as a child. Remember those days where the only care you had in the world was where you were going to go on your bike today?

Do you remember how wonderful it was to just play? It was great not to have an agenda or a plan, but to meet up with your friends and have fun. You found amazing ways to do this and make it exciting. You used your imagination and could make a stick anything you needed it to be. Well in this challenge you are going to revisit those days of your youth and bring it into your intimacy.

Many of you may recall having squirtgun battles with your friends or siblings. It was so refreshing and such fun to get outside on a hot day and blast each other with water. You could target people that you wanted to get back at without being mean. Heck, on the really hot days you wanted to be the one to get drenched. Well, now you are going to change up the desire in your squirtgun battle a little and make it more of an adult game.

You are going to take that same exhilaration and bring it to your intimacy. That youthful spirit and excitement is going to make you have a wonderful and romantic time. "This sounds crazy!" you might be thinking, but as you read how to complete this challenge I believe you will be chomping at the bit to get started.

Where to perform:

Obviously, you can't be running around your back yard playing an adult game like you would if you were having a squirtgun battle unless you happen to have a tall privacy fence or live out in a very rural neighborhood. However, doing it in the house is a little tricky also because you don't want to get stains on the carpet or furniture. So that leads to a couple of ideas that will get you out of the bedroom though.

The bathroom is usually a good place to start. Most bathrooms are designed to get a little wet and have flooring and wall covering made to handle liquids. The kitchen is another area that is made to be cleaned with hard surface floors and easily cleanable appliances. If neither of these places will work for you, then I suggest getting a drop cloth to lay down over you bed or wherever you will end up.

A quick word of caution - make sure you are safe in this challenge. With the supplies and the surfaces you will be standing on it might get a little slick. That means that you could take a hard fall if you slip – so be careful!! Oh, and try to keep your mouth shut during the saturation period. Lubrication in your mouth, especially a larger amount, might be unpleasant.

What you will need:

I suggest getting some cheap squirtguns at your local discount store. Don't get the really expensive ones because they most likely will get ruined in this process. Plus you want a "squirt" not a "waterfall" like some of those amazing new squirtguns can pack. The ones I am talking about should only cost a couple of dollars each. You will also need a thin lubricant. You cannot have a thick one because it will not work in the squirtgun. The lubricant has to be thin enough to flow easily through the workings of the squirt gun itself. If you can't find a lubricant that will work, you can grab some baby oil and it will be just fine. (I must caution you about baby oil though. It is not recommended as a lubrication for sexual activity – it can cause some women to get infections.) You also should grab some cheap swim goggles to protect your eyes from getting lubrication in them.

Protection for your house is another thing you have to look at. Lubrication and baby oil can stain. Make sure you cover up anything that could be ruined by a stain. Some lubes say they don't leave stains, but I still recommend taking precautions. You can pick up cheap drop cloths in the painting aisle of most stores. Take the time in advance to cover up things before you start that way you can enjoy the battle without concern of where your squirts are going.

How to complete:

Put your lube or oil inside your squirtgun. I recommend doing this over the sink so that any excess is easily washed down the drain. Make sure you have your goggles on. Now, it is time to strip down. You could wear a bathing suit if you like, but if you are inside, I suggest getting totally naked. That way you won't ruin your bathing suit.

Stand apart from each other at least five feet or so and get your squirtgun ready. Start at the same time. Choose who will say "begin" or "go". When the word is given to start, begin pumping your lubrication upon your lover. Make sure to take aim and soak down any area that might need extra lubrication. Aim for the breasts or nipples and make sure to give an extra few squirts to the genital area. Graciously unload the entire contents of your squirtgun onto your partner, and if you are the one whose gun runs out of ammo first, then you just have to wait and take it from your partner.

Another variation would be to take turns soaking each other down. Have one partner raise his/her hands as you soak him/her down with precision and accuracy. Once you unload your squirtgun it becomes the other partner's turn to do the shooting.

Once both partners have had their chance at being the target and the shooter it is time to meet in the middle to evaluate the damage. Push your bodies next to each other and enjoy the slick skin. Use you hands to rub in excess oil or just by rubbing your bodies together. View this as foreplay and make it last as long as you can. Once you both are lubed and ready it is time to make love. Be lighthearted and full of laughter as you enjoy this new twist to a childhood game.

Position Tracker

As sexual beings we have been amazed at the different positions for sex since the beginning of time. You can look back long ago and find interesting positions noted in books such as the Kama Sutra as well as ancient structures such as the Khajuraho Temples in India. These temples show us human fascination with sexual positions. The quest for these positions didn't die out - just go look in any bookstore today, and you can find countless books on sexual positions. Some are in great detail and some are comical in their approach. However, they all appeal to the quest to find all the different ways one can achieve intercourse with his/her partner.

Now, most of these publications seem to be geared toward heterosexual couples. You would obviously need different books for same sex couples. Many believe that changing the position in lovemaking will offer a different experience and make their sex life better.

Some of the positions you will find are impossible for the normal couple to get into. As you look through the options you likely realize that you need to be a contortionist to get into them. Can anyone really stand on his/her head and be able to achieve orgasm? Maybe – maybe not. Instead of just focusing on what positions to try you need to consider which positions seem possible to you and your partner.

This challenge is to help you start to figure out and challenge yourself to find all the positions that you can achieve during your sexual intimacy. Wading through all the books and online resources will be the challenge to get to the fun part of trying them out. With a little studying and ingenuity the sky is the limit on what you can try. As you go into this challenge make sure you consult your medical professional to ensure you are healthy enough for such activities.

You will most likely find some positions that you will like to revisit from time to time. Not only is this a wonderful addition to your challenges' library, but it also will be the one challenge that you can stretch out as long as you like.

Where to perform:

This challenge can and will be performed in many different places. Unlike most this challenge will take you several different lovemaking sessions. The nature of the positions you choose to partake of will determine where you will perform each session. You might encounter a position that requires you to stand up or one that might require the use of a chair. To tell you exactly where you will be making love during this challenge is impossible so you can skip on down to the next section and get closer to starting your challenge.

What you will need:

You will need a wide range of sexual positions. You can go to the bookstore and pickup several books on the subject or you can start searching the Internet and print out as many positions as you can find. There are several sexual position websites on the net that will help you with this challenge. After you gather as many positions as you can find, you will need to gather the items you normally use doing sex. Things like condoms, lubes or sex toys may be on your list. You might also need some extra props, as I will call them, so that you can achieve the positions. For example, you might need a stool or a chair to be able to achieve some positions. Some other positions might require the use of a large amount of pillows. You will just have to decide on your own what other items you need after you pick which positions you and your partner are going to try.

How to complete:

You need to connect with your partner and wade through all the positions you have collected. Take time to figure out which ones you want to try. One thing you have to remember is that this is a joint effort. It is important that you are both okay with the positions. You might want to try a position and your partner might say, "No way!" If this happens, you have two options. The first one is to absolutely forget about it. The second option might be to bargain for it. Say for example you want this position and your partner doesn't. Yet, a little farther into your search you find one that your partner wants to try and you don't. Well, maybe you can make an agreement to try his/hers if he/she tries yours? Of course, it is very important to respect your partner's wishes. If he/she is not comfortable with a position and will not agree to try it, do not push him/her. Let it go and move on.

Set a number of positions you want to try and then pick that number of positions from your books, Internet research or other media. Make a chart with them on it. It can be a simple word chart with the names of each position. Or, you might want to be creative and make a wonderful picture chart of the positions. You can mark them out as you achieve or attempt them. Keep a record and once you achieve or attempt all of them reward your relationship in some manner. Maybe you could take a trip or reward yourselves with a new sex toy. You set the standards and the reward.

This can be fun and exciting. You will start looking for new things to try and take your sexual relationship to the next level. The beauty of this challenge is that you can do it over and over again and have a different outcome each time. Since you will probably never be able to try every position thought up by our human counterparts this challenge could possibly last you a lifetime. Heck, it might even be a reason for you to get into better shape.

Cell Phone Erotica

Okay this challenge is going to give in to technology. Nowadays almost everyone has a cell phone. In fact, many people no longer have a landline. This technology has led to some very interesting advances in our daily living and how we communicate with one another.

Have you ever been hoping that your partner will be turned on when you get home from a long day at work? Maybe you are the one hoping that your partner will come home and sweep you off your feet and make passionate love to you. We can sit and hope that he/she is thinking about us in a sexy way or we can help the situation out a little.

One thing about this challenge is that it has some problems. Once it starts there is a huge jump in people leaving work early and burning up vacation time. Also, there are tasks at home not getting completed as couples are not wasting any time and leaving no time for chores. As you start this challenge understand it will get you hot and very excited. You will suddenly find yourself wanting to rip the clothes off your partner and make love in a ferocious manner.

Where to perform:

This will take place in many different places. However, the ending place should be where the two of you can interact freely and passionately. Hopefully, you will be able to make it into the safety of your home before the mood hits you too strongly. In the beginning, you will be performing this challenge anywhere you might happen to be with your cell phone. It could be at work, at the park, or even at your kid's baseball game. Please note that you should NOT do this while driving though. If you are at work, make sure you are not violating any work policies that might get you fired. You also want to make sure that other people will not have your cell phone or have access to it, because they might not understand.

What you will need:

Obviously, you need a cell phone and the ability to send and receive text messages. If you don't have a cell phone, you have some other options. You could use an email system by adapting this into an email erotic exchange. If you are really old school and are so against technology that you don't have a computer or a cell phone, you could use a notepad or journal to pass back and forth between the two of you. Other than the above-mentioned items, the only other things you will need are what you would normally use during sexual intimacy with your partner. Birth control, lubes, toys are a few that you might use.

How to complete:

You will be using the texting feature on your cell phone to get your partner turned on. The fun part is it works both ways as you are trying to turn your partner on he/she is trying to do the same to you. Doing this back and forth is an extremely entertaining and fun way to get aroused. You need to choose a day to do this challenge and you may even want to choose who is going to start this erotic texting. Then you must both agree to take turns texting with the understanding that sometimes you might have to wait a while for a response. Lastly, just like when you are making love you want to make it last as long as you can. Don't start out too quickly. Avoid premature texting.

You have laid the groundwork, and you are ready to start. The partner, who was chosen to go first, will type the start to an erotic story into his/her cell phone and send it to the other partner. Upon receiving the message the other partner will put in the next part of the story and text it back. This will continue until you both can return home to live out the sexy text message erotic story you have created. I suggest each partner texts a sentence or two during each text message. Don't make your texts too long. Be ready because things might not go exactly as planned. I also suggest making up fake names and not using your own just in case someone finds your phone and reads your messages.

Below is a sample of how this challenge might work.

TEXT #1 - "It was a hot day in Texas, so hot that even the pool Suzy was sitting by felt like bath water."

TEXT #2 -"Suzy pulled an ice cube from her drink and slowly worked it around her chest to feel it's cool wet touch"

TEXT #3 - "Suzy's nipples were obviously enjoying the ice as they stood at attention to hopefully attract the ice cube."

TEXT #4 - "John stood on the other side of the pool and felt his himself start to become hard…"

TEXT #5 - "Suzy saw John watching and became more adventures with the ice."

TEXT #6 - "Suzy slowly slid the ice into her bikini bottoms and moaned as the ice turned to water as it touched her."

You are hopefully starting to get the picture here. As mentioned above, if you can't achieve this challenge with a cell phone, you can use email or even pass a tablet back and forth between the two of you.

The beauty of this is that you can do it over and over and it will never turn out the same. It also can give hints to your lover of what you would like him/her to do to you or have you do to him/her. You can even use it as foreplay so that you are both ready to attack one other when you finally meet up. The important part is to make the story hot and sexy one sentence at a time.

The Sexual Bucket List

Most of us have heard of a bucket list. A bucket list is a list of things you want to accomplish before you leave this lifetime. It can be a group of places you want to venture to or a listing of activities you want to partake in before you draw your last breath. It seems like the older we get the more important these items on our bucket list become. That is one reason you see older people skydiving or going on exotic trips. They have more time and become more focused on their bucket list. They are also saying, "I am getting the most out of my life."

Why can't you start a sexual bucket list of things you want to do before you pass away or are unable to perform them? You might be thinking, "Well, this list is going to be pretty short." If so, then maybe you will want to consider some new options. There is a whole world out there of exciting sexual experiences you can share with your lover. In fact, you don't even have to get too far out of your comfort zone to experience them. You can create a sexual bucket list that will keep you and your partner busy and happy for the rest of your lives.

Half of the excitement of the challenge is planning out how to accomplish these feats together.

Where to perform:

I suggest sitting down at the table or desk to have your original brainstorming session on what to put on your list. You might want to be near your computer or have books available to search for interesting ideas to add to the list. You could even relax in your bed while you discuss things to add.

What you will need:

You will need a notebook and a pen. As mentioned above, a computer with Internet access or books would be helpful. Find some good websites and or catalogs with a wide selection of adult toys to choose from. Travel brochures might also be helpful in choosing items to put on your list. This might sound a little odd, but you might even want to get a bucket as a symbolic way to keep your list. Use it to store you notebook or you could put your ideas on little slips of paper and throw them in the actual bucket to be drawn out when the time arises.

How to Complete:

Start by compiling a list of all the sexual adventures you would like to try and the places around the world you would like to make love with your partner. Write down everything that comes to your mind on the notebook as a way to remember these beautiful and wonderful ideas. As you both throw out ideas you might find out some interesting things about your partner. Heck, you might even find that both of you would love to try the same thing, but you had both been too shy or afraid of what your partner might think to bring it up. Do not worry about filling out your entire bucket list in one sitting. Just write down all you can think of at the time. Other things will come to you later and you can always go back and put them on the list.

An interesting and fun idea is to try and add a new item to the list each time you complete one of the other items. You need to keep refreshing this list as a dedication to keep living life with a sexual flair. You might put the same thing back on the list after you complete it. If it was fun and exciting, why not do it a second time? Don't worry about your list growing too large. This offers you numerous opportunities to keep your sex life from becoming mundane.

Below are some suggestions of things someone might have on his/her sexual bucket list. The selection below shows how simple or how detailed your list can become. Use it as a guide and then get ready to have the time of your life.

Sexual Bucket List Suggestions

Oral sex outside

Make love in a pool

Engaging in anal play

Make love in India

Find a secluded place to make love during a family function

Make love 10 days in a row

See how many times you can make love in a day

Visit Stonehenge, soak up the energy, and make love nearby

Dressing up for specific role-play

Try some light bondage

Take Tantric workshop

Try a new position every month

Make love on the kitchen table

Go to a hotel for a couple of hours to make love

Try a new Sexy Challenge every month

Etc.

Start out slowly and put a couple of things on your list that will be easy to achieve. This way the list stays in your mind. If you put too many challenging things on the list, it might be a year or so before you can achieve any of them. I suggest mixing it up and putting something not so grand on your list every once in a while to keep the list moving. You will experience a sense of accomplishment as you mark things off your list – not to mention the pleasure you will experience and the fact that the bond between you and your partner will deepen and strengthen.

Mixing it up

This challenge will have you mixing things up. Putting more effort into foreplay and taking your time before actually getting into the act of making love. Each of you will get to experience sensations as your body starts to desire more and more touch. Building your excitement into a frenzy. This is great for those that love a great long loving experience. Way too often we rush through the early stages of intimacy to get closer to the end result. Why not stretch it out by mixing things up a little bit?

Make sure you set a good amount of time aside for this challenge. People who love foreplay and teasing will melt when presented with this adventure. Forcing both partners to slow down a little while having to change things up a bit is something many experts suggest. Getting excited already? That is the point.

What you will need:

You will need some sort of time keeping device. Be it a stopwatch or a clock - anything that you can quickly look at during your intimacy. Many cell phones have alarms you can set, so you could actually use your cell phone. Other than that the other items you need would be the items you normally use during your lovemaking. Things like birth control, toys, lubes, etc. I am sure you know what things you use and are comfortable with so I won't go into anymore detail on that.

Where to perform:

Obviously you will need a private place where you can both feel comfortable for an extended period of time. Your bedroom is the best suggestion. However, you could perform it anywhere that you can avoid interruptions. Make sure wherever you decide upon you have easy access to any items you would use during intimacy. I would also suggest having many pillows in the area to aid in this challenge.

How to complete:

First, get all your supplies ready and close to your intimate area. Make sure they are within arm's length of you and on a sturdy structure so that you don't lose them during the events to come. Next, make a nest out of all the pillows placing them around the area for quick additions to the festivities. Place your time keeping device where you can see it easily or hear the alarm when it sounds. Make a mental inventory of all the things that the two of you normally do during your intimate encounters. Now throw them out the window. Not really, but I want to break away from the normal here and get some new excitement flowing. Think of things you want to try or positions you want to give a whirl, or different ways to stimulate your partner.

On your timing device set it to go off every five minutes or make a note of the time on the clock and five minute intervals. Start by kissing each other softly and then more passionately. When the alarm goes off or you reach the five-minute mark it is time to mix it up. Change what you are doing and enter into a different way to stimulate your partner. Maybe for the next five minutes you both flip around and rub or caress each other's feet stroking the calves of your mate while he/she does the same to you. Then when the five-minute mark hits again, move to something else such as playing with each other's nipples stroking, licking, pinching them to heighten arousal. Continue on with this process of mixing things up every five minutes. Sure it might be disappointing if something is feeling really good, but you can always come back to it in another time frame. This sounds simple enough, but I want to challenge you to avoid all normal routines even to the point of abandoning your normal position for sex. For most heterosexual couples that will be the missionary position.

Even when you start with the actual intercourse I want you to mix it up every five minutes or less. This will allow you to hopefully experience several different positions during one intimate evening. Not only is this a great way to change up the pace, but you might actually find something that really works for the two of you. The amazing beauty of this challenge is that you can do it over and over again without it ever being the same. How much fun is that to have in your sex life?

You can hit many different angles and have many different experiences with this loving adventure. Switching every five minutes helps you touch on many different experiences. For example you can experience toys, oral sex, kissing, extended foreplay, teasing, light bondage, etc. all in one session. The amazing part is how long it will last. You could go on for hours. Of course, don't deny yourself or your partner. Set up a code word to speak when you crave to finally orgasm. Shout it out loud and clear when you want and need that energy pulsating through your body.

A variation to this challenge is that you could allow each partner to take turns and give instructions to the other. This gives more control of what happens pleasure-wise to the partner receiving the pleasure. It is great as long as you both get a chance to give the instructions and feel the pleasure. If you don't feel comfortable verbally giving instructions write them down and throw them in a hat to be drawn out by your lover. That will really mix things up because you won't have any idea what order these pleasures will come to you.

Use your imagination to make this a fun and exciting experience. You could also check out books on sexual positions or different foreplay techniques to help you experience new and powerful intimacy.

Butter Up Your Love

Featuring Sex Butter

This challenge is based on a wonderful product that not only improves the actual sex act, but it is also good for your body and the environment. Wow, what a combination! You might be wondering what this amazing product is. Well, the name of this magickal elixir is Sex Butter. This challenge was a bit of a challenge in of itself to write simply because this amazing product seems to speak for itself. Are you wondering what makes this lubrication unique and why it stands out from others? Well, here is why directly from www.sexbutter.net...

What You Want to Know About Sex Butter...Sex Butter is 100% organic oils, safe, hormone-free, paraben-free, chemical-free, and hypo-allergenic. Sex Butter has no known drug interactions. After applying Sex Butter, it takes minutes to feel the sensation begin and may last up to an hour. This product may be reapplied at anytime during foreplay or intercourse. Sex Butter was specifically formulated in the high altitude clean mountain air of New Mexico straight from the alchemist's apothecary. The butter is formulated not only to be fun but also very functional in aiding, healing and protecting the skin.

How Sex Butter can work for you…*Sex Butter allows women to feel intense pleasure easily and effortlessly. The special blend of 100% organic essential oils helps to create heightened sensation during foreplay as well as intercourse. Sex Butter lubricates allowing everlasting sexual pleasure. Some of the general feedback we got from women during testing:*

Heightened sensation overall during foreplay and intercourse

Increased number of orgasms

More intense orgasms – with internal and external stimulation

Increased overall lube or lubrication

Freedom from painful sex

Greater endurance

Overall feeling of satisfaction from the whole experience

We gave Sex Butter to women ranging from 25-70 including:

Women going through perimenopause

Women in menopause

Women taking all kinds of medication

Women post hysterectomy

Cancer patients in remission

Cancer patients taking chemotherapy

Women who tested Sex Butter have found Sex Butter extremely effective at boosting sexual appetite, arousal, sensation, and fulfillment. Men love Sex Butter too! Why? Great lubrication, wonderful sensation during foreplay and intercourse, quicker recovery time, sensations even after the experience, and their women were fully satisfied and happy.

I have had the pleasure of working with many lubes in my time! Sex Butter, however, stands out as the "cream of the crop". I am excited to tell you that I found Sex Butter gets better the longer you use it. It is, also, safe for your skin – inside and out. It is edible and 100% natural. Heck, our food isn't that safe. With Sex Butter you can apply lube and still kiss, lick, suck any part of the body without having to worry about a nasty taste in your mouth. Plus, even though you likely won't be thinking about the environment during your passionate time together, you will be doing it a wondrous favor. Mmm, I also must mention the amazing chocolate mint aroma that Sex Butter offers you – it is sexy too. Enough of the chitchat it is time to get on to the Sexy Challenge.

Within this challenge you will be using the wonderful properties of Sex Butter to connect with your partner in many ways. Touch is an outstanding gift we as humans are allowed to enjoy, but many of us don't use it enough. I am inviting you to touch each other in numerous and sensual ways. I suggest you allow plenty of time for this challenge as the butter gets better and better the longer you use it, and this could possibly be the most fun you have had in bed in a long time.

Where to perform:

This challenge is multidimensional and you can perform it anywhere you normally have sex: the bedroom, the couch, or even the kitchen table – after all Sex Butter *is* edible and it doesn't stain. If you want to branch out a little, keep your butter in various places around the house so you will always be prepared when the moment arises. Put it in your desk drawer for a romantic lunch or maybe in the glove box of your car or even keep a jar of it in your handbag for those spontaneous moments. You might even keep it in your overnight bag for when you and your lover have a chance to get away.

What you will need:

Obviously, I suggest you have Sex Butter, but basically that is it! (You might want to have two jars available – one for each of you. Plus, you don't want to run out. TRUST ME!) You can use any other items, which you normally bring into your intimacy, but now they will come with the enhancement of this amazing butter. Once you give it a try, I venture to say you will be hooked.

How to complete:

For starters, set the mood for a long and enjoyable evening. Light a few candles or set the lighting low so that you can see each other just enough and enjoy the shadows playing off of your bodies. If you enjoy music, put a little music on. Keep it low so that you can hear the sounds that tell you your partner is enjoying what you are doing. Make sure you have your Sex Butter within reach as well as any other items you might be using for this challenge. Remove all the unnecessary clothing and let the soft light caress you both.

Start by running your hands over each other's bodies. See how the skin of your partner feels under your touch. Taste his/her skin as you place light, feathery kisses in the places that he/she loves to be kissed. Go slowly and enjoy the sensations as you touch as many parts of the body as you can. Use light and gentle touch as you stroke the legs and arms. Venture to your partner's back and lightly touch or scratch in long smooth strokes. Avoid the genitals at this point. You want to extend the enjoyment of this challenge. All this is priming the skin to receive the gift of the butter.

Once both of you have enjoyed the sensations of feeling each other's bare skin, it is time to change up that feeling by adding the butter. Take small amounts and apply it to different areas of your partner's body – a little goes a long way. Again, avoid the genitals – that enjoyment will come soon. For now, rub it on your partner's forearms, thighs, feet, forehead, lips etc. – anywhere that might get missed during your normal sexual experience.

Here is the sensual and sexy kicker; you need to find a way to apply it onto his/her skin without using your hands!! You can use your face, your forearms, thighs, feet, chest/breasts, or stomach. Heck, you can even use your rear end if you like. This will connect you and your partner in ways that you have never connected before. I still want you to avoid using the genitals – just for now. I know, I am teasing you. It will all be worth it in the end. Spend a good amount of time taking turns and doing this to each other. During this time focus on how differently your partner feels with the silky smooth Sex Butter upon his/her skin. This phenomenal lubrication helps bring forth one's natural pheromones.

165

Smell the amazing difference as your partner's personal, natural scent mixes with the tantalizing smell of the butter. At this point, you have transformed your partner into a Goddess/God of sensual pleasure.

It is time for things to get a little more heated. Pick some areas on your partner's body to put the butter by using your genitals.

Men you can place it between the cheeks of your partner's rear end and massage it in with your penis. You can put some on his/her chest and allow your penis to slip and slide all over this erogenous zone. Be creative – another idea might be that you put some in his/her armpit and allow your penis to explore a new place on your partner's body.

Ladies this is a great sensation for you too. This puts you in control of your pleasure. Put some on your partner's thigh and massage it in with your vulva. Enjoy the up and down stroking. This will open your lotus of pleasure. Put some on the tip of your partner's nose and use it as your personal sex toy. Again, be creative – flip your partner over and put a bit at the base of his/her spine. Use that area of fleshy firmness to massage all the areas of pleasure between your legs. Thrust yourself deep into it and experience the sensation on your clitoris. Your partner will love how use his/her body to pleasure yourself. Here's an exciting little tip: Apply a small dab of Sex Butter to your G-spot. This will enhance your experience even further and get you out of you head and into your body. Isn't it getting hot in here?

Okay, now time for the tasting. If needed, apply some to your partner's genitals and gently bite, lick, and suck until you see that he/she is obviously aroused. At this point you can take your lover to climax orally or you can back off and let him/her simmer a bit longer.

No matter how you choose to enjoy this adventure (orally, anally, vaginally or by hand) you will be able to do so with passionate intensity and speed or you can choose to do so slowly and methodically.

After this fun evening of amazing intimate play and heightened sensations you will be singing the praises of Sex Butter to your friends and maybe even strangers on the street! This excitement is because you have found the Holy Grail of sexual lubrication. Thank you for buttering up with us. Oh, by the way Sex Butter is fantastic when you are alone or with a "toyfriend" (wink, wink)!!!

Mummify Me

Okay, so at the time of the writing of this challenge it is Halloween time. People are out in their costumes running around scaring each other and asking for candy. As a couple you might be tired of the regular old sexy costumes. I mean how many times can a guy wear a loincloth and a woman be a sexy vampire. We have to look a little deeper to find a costume that not only can make us feel sexy, but create a passion filled sexy challenge.

One of the sexiest times in history to me was ancient Egypt with the heavy eye make-up and the small amount of clothing that they wore. When we think about ancient Egypt and Halloween there is one thing that pops into our minds. Mummies! This just might have been the single most mysterious element from the time of the pharos. Was there a connection for mummies and the afterlife? Did they go to the place where they could live life again? We will never know that for sure in this lifetime.

The point is Egypt and Mummies are sexy! Well, if you don't think so now, you will change your mind after you enjoy this challenge. Close your eyes and let yourself wander back in time. Feel the sand of the great desert and beauty of the Sphinx and Great Pyramid and get set to shriek in horror or in your case ecstasy at the image of the mummy coming towards you.

Where to perform:

I suggest you perform this at your home - in the comfort of your bedroom or another place that you can take the time to dress up. More important than where might be when to do it. Obviously, around Halloween time would be a wonderful time for this spooky challenge. However, any time there is a full moon would be an interesting time too. The moon has many magical powers and reaches far beyond the horror movies that bring out the werewolves.

What you will need:

Toilet paper is the biggest part of this challenge. You will need plenty of it and I suggest getting the higher quality. You will also need anything you normally use during a sensual sexual encounter with your partner. Condoms, lubes, and toys are all common items within people's sex lives so bring them. Other optional things you might want to bring would be things that might help set the mood of ancient Egypt. Thinks like sandals, bangles and bracelets, or even just some hieroglyphics drawn and placed on the wall. Candles are also a nice touch to give the feeling of the torches that would rest on the walls of the tomb of the mummy.

How to complete:

Start the evening by bathing or showering using your favorite soaps and oils. Both of you clean yourself well and then when you get out of the shower or bath make sure to dry yourself off to the best of your ability. Take some time and let yourself dry even more. Relax a little in your naked state. Once you both are bathed and dry it is time to start this ancient tradition of mummification. Get your toilet paper out and begin wrapping each other up. Make sure you do it in a manner so that you can both move. Wrapping the legs together will only lead to falls and the inability to approach each other. That is not what you want on this night. Cover as much of the body as you can, take your time and use a lot of toilet paper. The only parts you need to leave exposed are the eyes and the mouth. This is so you can see and speak.

Once you are both mummified it is time to approach each other in a sensual and inviting way. Kiss each other passionately and feel the connection through the toilet paper. Feel the passion that is only kept out from the paper between the two of you. Make your way over to the bed and continue the mummy make-out session. Notice the changes in your mummy partner. Is his erection breaking through his makeshift bandages, are her juicy lady parts helping to remove these bandages from sensual areas. Can you see your partner's hardened nipples protruding through the wrap? Once you both feel the time is right you need to make the sacrifice of love to each other.

Here is what I want you to do at this point. I want you to try to keep as much toilet paper on both your bodies as possible. Another rule is you cannot remove any of the wrap with your hands. Most of the wrap will finally fall off and you will be left with a mummy that has been transformed into an Egyptian Prince or Princess.

Some variations you might try are just wrapping up one of you and the other partner becomes the sacrificial offering to the mummy. Let the mummy have its way with you, as you are its personal love slave for this evening. Another thing you might try is to lay the mummy down on the bed and let the other partner slowly start removing the wrapping of the mummy in a slow and sensual manner. Find some Egyptian music to play in the background for added effects. Or, if you really want to get a bit crazy, try wrapping yourselves up into one mummy. Just be careful and have all things out of the way as you could possibly fall. To really set the mood, have an Egyptian style dinner complete with wine.

The point is to bring some fireworks into your intimacy and with this mummified experience you can preserve the memory for a long long time.

Confetti Kisses

This challenge is a celebration of your love for each other. Have you ever been to a parade? People are cheering and the air buzzes with excited energy as a multitude of colorful confetti and streamers fill the sky.

Why shouldn't you bring that type of excitement and enthusiasm into your intimacy? Each time you get a chance to enjoy your partner it should be a celebration. I'm not suggesting that you form a parade each time the two of you want to be intimate with each other, but it should still be a celebration between the two of you. This will help you experience your intimate play as a celebration.

Where to Perform:

You will probably want to do this one at home. You might create a bit of a mess and even though it will be colorful and playful disorder it might be better to have it home where you can pick it up without questioning eyes. Your bedroom should work nicely for this celebration. You might consider using other areas of your home, but you must take into account whether or not you have children or guests over. A nice touch for this challenge I will talk about later is having a room with a ceiling fan.

What you will need:

The main thing you will need is confetti. You can go out and purchase some at your local store or you can make your own out of tissue paper. The choice is up to you. I suggest getting confetti that is a little larger in size. There are two reasons for this: 1) It will be easier to clean up after the celebration 2) If the confetti is too small it will make it difficult to enjoy this challenge. Other things you might want to have are a recording of a crowd cheering and sunglasses to protect your eyes from confetti falling in them. *You can substitute something in place of the confetti if you would like. Flower petals are one other option.

How to complete:

To start with make the decision as to which one of you will go first. That person will strip down to the least amount of clothing that he/she feels comfortable with. Of course, I suggest doing this naked, but that is up to you. He/she will lie down on the bed, sofa, or floor and close his/her eyes or slip on the above-mentioned sunglasses to avoid confetti getting in the eyes. This would be the time to play the cheering crowd audio if you located one. Put a little confetti in your hand and gently blow it across your partner's body. Watch it fall onto various parts of your partner.

You could also consider sprinkling the confetti over your partner or a favorite of mine is to place the confetti on a ceiling fan. When you are ready, you turn the fan on low. You and your partner will be transferred into a gentle whirlwind of colorful confetti. It truly becomes an amazing show as you watch the confetti gently landing upon his/her body.

The next step involves each spot on your partner's body where confetti landed. Remove each piece of confetti and replace it with a kiss. You decide what kind of kiss that body part gets. You might consider a few light feathery kisses as well as long wet kisses. Varying the types of kisses adds to this challenge, as your partner will not know what to expect next. Once you have kissed away all the confetti on your partner it is time to switch it up. Trade spots so you become the receiver of drifting confetti and your partner the confetti thrower, blower, or sprinkler.

Once you have both completed a round of confetti kisses you will probably be ready to move on to more passionate lovemaking. Mmmm...enjoy your intimate play and celebration and your finale of "fireworks".

Message in a Bottle
Quickie

Entice your lover as if you were on a deserted island or a pirate searching for treasure. All you need is a bottle & a piece of paper. Write a short request on the paper. For example: "How about joining me on Pleasure Island?" "Rescue me & I will give you my treasure," or "Argh Matey, How about giving up the booty?" Roll the message up & put it inside the bottle. Leave part of it sticking out the top so your lover can retrieve it. Then float your bottle somewhere that he/she will find it: bathtub, sink, anything that holds water. Once the message is found the fun on your "deserted island" will heat up.

Trading Panties

This sexy challenge is meant to get the two of you out of your comfort zone. You are going to go to a public place to complete this challenge. The beauty of it is that no one besides the two of you will know it is happening. This challenge will get your blood pumping and afterwards you will say, "I can't believe we did that." This activity will create giggles and secretive smiles that others will wonder about. If you feel a bit nervous about completing this challenge, don't worry. By the time it is done the two of you will have created a new bond. What is even more enticing is that by the end of this challenge the two of you will be ready to race home and reward each other in a sensual and passionate way.

Where to perform:

This challenge will take place in a restaurant that you can sit down and eat your meal. It can be a fancy restaurant or it can be a fast food place. I suggest a fancier restaurant if at all possible. In choosing the restaurant, you might want to consider restaurants that are located a bit away from where you live. You might consider going to a near-by town or make a weekend out of it and take a romantic little trip somewhere. Either way you want to pick a restaurant you don't frequent often – unless you are really brazen.

What you will need:

Besides money to pay for your meal the only other thing you will both need is underwear. I assume you both have some at home to use. If you like, feel free to go out and purchase a new pair just for this occasion. If you want to make the evening even more interesting, you can pick out underwear that is very gender specific. Some ideas include: thongs, tighty whities, crotchless or g-strings.

How to complete:

Make sure the two of you have on the underpants you have selected. After you are seated in the restaurant you may begin the challenge.

One of you goes to the restroom first and removes your underpants. You then bundle them up and hide them in your pocket or purse so they will not get noticed. Then return to your table and casually slip them to your partner. At this point your partner excuses himself/herself to go to the restroom. Inside the restroom he/she slips out of his/her own underpants and slips on the other ones. Return to the table with the undies out of sight and pass them to the first partner. The first partner will then return to the restroom and put on those underwear. Once both of you have switched your underpants/panties, you return to the table and enjoy the wonderful meal before you. Everyone in the building except the two of you will be unaware of the mission you just completed. The hard part is not to start laughing or smiling when the two of you look at each other. Once you have finished eating, simply pay the bill, leave a tip and head for home.

Upon arriving home you both must prove to the other you have completed the task by stripping down to your underpants. Once you quit laughing at each other it is time for the reward. Begin passionately kissing each other while you still have the other partner's underpants on. Make sure to run your hands over each other's new underpants and say how sexy they look. Finish the evening by making passionate love to each other. You will both be laughing in the morning as you pick the underpants up off the floor. The beauty of this is that only the two of you will know. It is your secret. Plus, each time you see those garments in the wash you will remember your fun and exciting evening.

Let me share some variations you might add to this. If the size of the partners makes it impossible for you to actually wear each other's underpants or if it is just a little too far out of your comfort zone, here is a suggestion. You can both just remove your underpants and return to the table of the restaurant finishing the meal commando. Slip your underpants to the your partner as proof. Whichever way you choose to proceed with this challenge you will get a good laugh and hopefully, a fascinating lovemaking session later.

Grocery Store Games

Okay, I know you are all thinking I am nuts. How can you possibly make grocery shopping an intimate experience? Well, I truly believe that you can make any experience intimate and romantic. It just depends on how you approach it. Grocery shopping is one that was a little bit difficult, but I managed to find a way, and I am going to present it to you in this challenge. No, you are not going to have to go make out in the fresh fruit section or venture into the frozen food section to get your nipples erect. The grocery store in this challenge is just the start to an event in the making.

When we shop together we usually stay together and stay on task. Our usual goal is to get in and out as quickly as possible. That is great for shopping, but it really sucks for intimacy. Who wants it to be over as quickly as possible? NOT ME! Now you might not think of spending time in the grocery store as foreplay, but this challenge might just change your mind on the subject. Orgasmic grocery shopping is one way to look at these suggestions and ideas. You likely will not be able to look at the grocery store in the same way again.

We all need to eat - that is a certainty. So, we have to go to the grocery store as a means of survival. Unless you are one of those rare people that can support yourself from your own land or can afford for someone else to do your shopping. We also need great sex in our relationship to have a fulfilling and passionate life. Why not combine these two events into something special for your relationship?

Where to perform:

Obviously, you are going to go to your local supermarket or shopping complex for the first part of this challenge. I consider this your "shop-olympics" part of the challenge. The second part will be the medal ceremony and this will need to be in a more private setting. Most likely you will be presenting the medals at your home and in your bedroom.

What you will need:

The basic things you will need are a grocery list, paper to write on, and money to pay for the items you will be purchasing. An optional item you might need is a camera - be it on your cell phone or an actual camera. You might also want a time keeping device – one for each of you.

How to complete:

As mentioned earlier, consider this as a shop-olympics complete with a medal ceremony for the gold medalist. Second place or silver medalist will get rewarded with the simple act of intimacy itself. The first thing you both need to do is decide on what sexual favor you want from your partner if you are the gold medalist. It could be oral sex or having your partner wear something sexy for you. It could even be a sensual massage. The choice is yours. Once you have the prizes decided upon it is time to go to the events. You could even make up little fake gold medals with your sexual favor listed on the back to be presented at the awards ceremony later in your bedroom.

The shop-olympics will consist of three events and be worth 1 point each. The person that wins 2 events or gets 2 points is the gold medalist and will receive their sexual gratification later. While this is a competition I like to think there are no losers, as you both will get to reap the rewards of intimacy after the events are complete. So, play fair and don't cheat. Let this be a fun and enjoyable activity for both of you. If you are one of those competitive people that cannot stand to lose at any cost, you need to just chill out and get over yourself. This is for love and romance not domination!

Your first event is a timed event. You both need to decide on a time frame such as 15 minutes to a half hour. You could go longer, but that might make this event boring. Once the time is determined you will both need a note pad or a camera and venture out to the store. What you are going to do is take pictures or write down items that remind you of your partner's sexy parts. For example, if your partner is a female you could take pictures of oranges that remind you of her breasts. If your partner is a male, then bananas and hot dogs are very obvious items that would remind you of his sexy parts. Either write them down or take a picture of each item as you see it. Then meet at the front of the store once time is up. Make a penalty for if you arrive late to the front of the store to avoid cheating. Be prepared to defend your choices and explain why you chose them. The winner and receiver of one point is the person that has the most pictures or items on his/her list.

The second portion of the shop-olympics is the speed event. Pick out 10 items and put them on a list. They can be the same 10 items or you can pick 10 items for your partner to find and he/she can pick 10 items for you to find. Make a starting and ending point somewhere in the store. Position yourselves at the starting line and get ready. One of you says go and you are both on your way. The one of you who returns the quickest back to the start/finish line with all 10 items is the winner and the one that receives the one point. At this point the gold medalist might already be determined, but you will still want to complete this last event.

The last event is to find the most non-sexual sexy item. Condoms and lubes could be considered sexy, but your search is to find something that isn't supposed to be sexy. The packaging just makes it seem that way. Maybe it is the person on the box of cereal that looks as though he/she is having an orgasm while eating cereal. It could be the sucker at the front of the store that is shaped similarly to a penis. Be creative and again set a time limit so this doesn't drag on and on. When comparing your choices for this part of the challenge be objective and admit defeat if your partner out does you.

In the strange event of a tie I would consider both partners winners and give each one of you gold medals and the sexual actions associated with the gold medals. Once the winner is determined it is time to set up the medal ceremony. If you can't run right home and present your award, plan it for later in the evening when you can enjoy and take your time presenting the award. Remember those that win gold medals in the Olympics are treated like heroes upon their return home. Don't expect anything less here. You might even play your national anthem or a favorite song.

Never has grocery shopping been this fun. Your grocery shopping experiences from now on will be tame compared to this experience.

Personal Zen Garden

Your sexual life may be a very exciting and passionate place. However, every now and then it is good to slow it down and bring some peace and tranquility into the passion. That is the object of this challenge. I want to incorporate the peace and tranquility that goes into creating a powerful Zen garden into your intimate play. With a little practice you will begin to open your mind to more enjoyment and differences that will give you an entirely new outlook on your sexual experience.

Zen Gardens are Japanese in tradition. Other names for these include rock gardens or dry gardens. These gardens feature rocks or stones along with a limited amount of vegetation. They are commonly found near Zen temples of meditation and their main influence was that of Zen Buddhism. Where many gardens might have water in the form of streams or ponds running through them a Zen Garden is dry and replaces the water with sand or gravel. The Zen Garden is constantly tended so that it remains neat and perfect in appearance. The Zen priests rake the gravel or sand is raked into patterns. It reminds me of the rippling water or waves in the ocean. The raking is considered a meditation and calms the mind as it is performed. The large stones in the garden represent the mountains and the land.

The raking is performed around these objects much as the water would run around them in nature. A Zen garden represents the harmony that nature has.

Today, you don't have to travel to a Zen temple to find such a garden though. In fact, they have become quite popular. It is not uncommon to see a small replica of a Zen Garden on an executive's desk or in a park. This wonderful way to calm your mind has made its way into everyday life. This is a good thing as long as they are not just a novelty and are really used for the right purpose.

I hope that in this challenge you will not only receive the peace that goes along with caring for a Zen garden, but that you will give the peace to your partner also. Venturing into the peace and tranquil space before you make love to each other is a fabulous way to honor not only each other, but also your relationship. It is important to note that you can take what you learn here and apply it to other areas of your life too. May peace be the guide of your journey.

What you will need:

Find 3-5 rocks that are smaller than the size of your fist. Wash these with gentle soap – perhaps, even soap with a lovely scent. You might consider finding a small rake as well. There are various options for this, such as a tiny decorative rake or even a back scratcher. If necessary, you can use a fork or even your fingers.

Warm lighting and soft music or calming sounds like a trickling stream are also things you will need.

Where to perform:

Find a comfortable place. This place should include a comfortable spot for the receiver to lie down – a bed, sofa, or soft cushions on the floor. It should also allow you to easily move around his/her body so that you can touch every part of your partner. Privacy is another factor to consider because most likely you will want the person that is acting as the Zen garden to be totally nude.

How to complete:

Decide who will receive first. That person then lies facedown. The other person strategically places the freshly washed rocks upon the first partner. Using the tiny rake or your fingernails gently start to groom the skin around the objects. Make long and slow stokes up and down the back. When you meet a rock simply and slowly rake around it. Calm your mind as you feel the pleasure you are giving to the person lying down. You might be able to see the pattern your light scratching is doing on your partner. It should look like the groomed Zen Garden. (A word of caution here. Make sure your scratching is light. The experience should not become painful. The intent is for it to be relaxing to both of you. If the scratching is too much for the receiving partner, just use your fingertips.)

Continue around the body, moving the rocks to the areas you are focusing on. Once you do the back of your partner move the rocks to his/her legs, feet and buttocks. Once you have gone over the entire back area have your partner roll over and repeat the process on his/her front. Besides the rocks the front of your partner's body will have some objects of its own. The breasts and penis are a couple that come to mind. Work around these areas as is if they were rocks also. If your partner likes, you can gently rake them too. Once you have completed your entire lover's body it is time to switch. Each of you will get to experience the calm serenity that is accompanied with giving and receiving.

At this point, you both rise and join in the middle of the bed or floor. You then embrace each other blending your naked bodies together. Then both of you slide your hand to the back of your partner and again start lightly raking each other's back at the same time. Let your lips meet in a kiss and close your eyes. Feel your freshly raked skin as it touches your partner's. Let your senses come alive with sensuality. Slowly move all of this Zen to a spot so that you may make love to each other. Start out slowly. Then, let your passion decide the pace. Keep things slow and sensual or if your passion is climbing allow it to rage like the power of the ocean. Once both partners have climaxed or gotten their fill of the passion lie together closely and return to raking each other's skin as you drift off.

Bang a Gong

Most people believe that a gong is just a musical instrument that adds exclamation to a musical arrangement. It is true that they are that, but they are so much more. While gongs have been used as a musical instrument throughout history they were usually used more as a signal than as part of a musical performance. It seems the origins of the gong come from China and can be traced back as far as 2000 B.C. They were used in religious ceremonies as well as weddings and festivals to mark the occasion as a special event. They could also be used to announce the approach of royalty or to summon attention for important speeches.

Gongs have even been used by our modern society in many different forms of entertainment. John Belushi used one in his skit on *Saturday Night Live* - Samurai Delicatessen to signal when the next order was ready. The band T.Rex produced a song called *Bang a Gong* on their 1971 album *Electric Warrior*. There was even a show called *The Gong Show* that aired during the 1970's. This show had people perform silly acts, and if they got gonged, they were kicked off the show. So, you see the gong has been with us for a long long time and used for a wide variety of things.

In this challenge, you are going to use it a little differently. You are going to use it as a signal to honor your relationship. The simple act of striking a gong will become part of your intimacy. You will soon feel the vibration the gong produces into your very soul. It is my hope that the gong will become a symbol of love and honor to you as well as the sound of passion. Get your mallets warmed up and get ready to introduce the gong into your relationship.

Where to perform:

This challenge will start in any room of the house you like. You can have your instrument set up in your bedroom, bathroom or living room for that matter. The sound should be able to travel through your house so that no matter where you are you will be able to hear it. I suggest setting the gong up in your bedroom to avoid having to leave the comfort of your love sanctuary to strike the gong. However, that is totally up to you.

What you will need:

You will need a gong of some sort for this challenge. It can be an official type of gong or a makeshift gong. There are many different types that you can find ranging in size from very large to very small. The sound they emit is also very different depending on the size and the material the gong is made of. Together try some out and see which one best fits into your price range and is appealing to both of you. Another option is to create your own gong. Items such as trashcan lids and drum cymbals work well too, but may not have the sacred feeling that a gong can have. You can use anything that makes a sound vibration. In fact, you might choose to use a singing bowl or a tuning fork. Whatever you choose to use, just make sure the sound is distinct and appealing to you and your partner.

How to complete:

The idea is to associate a sound vibration with a call or a completion. Introducing this sound to your intimate life will begin to allow you to associate the sound with pleasure and love. Releasing this sound will also be a sign to the powers that be (no matter what you believe) that you are honoring your relationship and passion. You have a couple of different paths this challenge can take. It can be a calling to lovers as what is about to happen or a signal of completion to the Universe. Because not only will this sound be heard by the two of you, but it will send its vibration out into the furthest reaches of the Universe. Plus, anyone within normal earshot will be aware of the sound, but they will not know the secret of the sound. That is only for the ones in the relationship to know.

Start by setting up your instrument in the desired location. Once set, the two of you need to discuss the intention of your message when you strike the gong. Will it be a call to make love or a signal that the two of you have shared one of the most beautiful pleasures within your life? You can do both if you wish. It is up to the two of you to choose and then commit to doing it.

If you choose to use the gong as a signal that you want to make love, you also need to put some rules in place. Decide on a timeframe in which you cannot strike the gong again. In other words, if you strike the gong and then you and your partner make love, perhaps, you will have the rule that you cannot strike it again for 48 hours. It is also important to allow one another to pass on lovemaking if he/she is simply not in the mood. Instead, perhaps you can spend some quiet time together – cuddling or at least holding hands. Now, you might also put into place that each of you are required to strike the gong at least once each week. (Remember this calls at the very least for cuddling or hand-holding.) Be certain you allow your partner time to respond. This should not be a call of immediate action. In fact, you might strike the gong in the morning before you leave for work with the anticipation of making love to your partner that evening.

If you choose to use the gong as a signal that the two of you just shared a passionate session of lovemaking, you still might want to add some rules. How many times will you strike the gong? Who will strike the gong? Will you strike it immediately or the following morning? Create your own rules in a way that you feel honors you both and your relationship.

No matter which path you choose, the two of you will find peace and harmony in the sound of the gong and it will lift your hearts whenever you need it to. Use it well and make it a ceremony that will last long into your relationship.

Test Your Limits

We have all heard the stereotype that men are always ready for sex. Well, this isn't always the case. Sometimes it is the women who can't get enough. The point is that we all have different sex drives. So there are a couple of questions: How can you tell which partner can handle the most intimacy? Can the one with the highest sex drive actually have more orgasms than the other partner?

The point of this challenge is to find out who can handle the most intimacy. Maybe once a day is enough for you. However, some people might desire it three times a day. It is all based on the individual.

You are going to push your partner to the limit and see how much intimacy he/she can truly handle. Some of you are out there jumping for joy right not thinking about this. Yet, I am willing to bet when this challenge is over, you won't have enough energy left for jumping up and down.

Make sure you are in good health prior to doing this challenge because it will test your physical endurance. Do not proceed unless you have checked with your doctor, and you are healthy enough for intense and multiple orgasms. I also suggest that you make sure you have plenty of water handy as sex can dehydrate your body. While this is designed to be fun, I want to encourage you to always be safe in your sexual pursuits. Safe sex is the best sex. And, "safe sex" means more than preventing pregnancy or STDs.

Where to perform:

Most likely your bedroom will be the best place. You want to make sure you are comfortable and that everything you need is easily accessible. Plus, you will probably be very tired at the end of this challenge. Being able to comfortably relax in your own bed will rank high on your list at this point.

What you will need:

Lubrication is an important part of this challenge. It will be important for both males and females. Any other items you would use during your normal sexual activity are a must. Condoms, sex toys, etc. are part of normal people's sex lives all over the world so bring them in and use them as intended. Some light bondage items to bind hands and feet would be helpful also. Towels are important for clean up too. Make sure you also bring a "safe word" with you. A safe word is a word or phrase you say to your partner, which tells him or her to stop immediately. This way there is no mistaking when you are done and/or can't take any more. Make this word something you don't normally say. Make it unique, but something you can both remember.

How to complete:

The goal is to see who can orgasm the most times in one day. I suggest using the whole day, but if you want to limit it to just a few hours that is up to the two of you. An important part of this challenge is to be honest with each other - no faking it. You can use any means necessary to achieve orgasm. You can use intercourse, oral sex, anal sex, masturbation, toys, vibrators, sleeves - the choice is up to you. Have something to keep track of your orgasms - a simple piece of paper and pen will do. However, if you want to go all out, maybe a huge chalkboard and a drum roll after each orgasm might be in order.

To kick off this challenge make love in the most normal way you do. Begin your day or session off right – then get even more creative. You might want to set an amount time between each lovemaking session – a time for recuperation. Don't expect your partner to have an amazing sexual experience with you then turn around and start right over again. Make sure to take time to eat and drink between sessions. It really is important to keep your energy up and to stay hydrated. Once you both feel rejuvenated, give it another try making sure to use enough lubrication. Chaffed skin will end this challenge very quickly. So, protect your delicate parts and use plenty of lubrication.

After the second round of sexual pleasure, take the time between and assess if you can proceed. Do not be ashamed if you decide you cannot continue. When one of you can't continue you may want to mix it up even more. At this point you can use sex toys to lead your partner to orgasm or you can use your hands to stimulate him/her to orgasm. Another option is that one or both of you masturbate. Remember to keep track of your orgasms. Obviously, the one who orgasms the most is the winner, not that you both didn't win, but you should have a reward for the master of the orgasm. Maybe the winner gets to decide where you are going to dinner the next night or maybe he/she chooses a place for you to take a short getaway.

It is possible that one of you will only be able to achieve one orgasm while the other achieves three or four. The important part is you both are enjoying each other as you orgasm or watch. And, after a full day or long session of love making, you are going to be relaxed and probably sleep quite well.

After a few months try this again to see if your numbers increase. Our sexual health is something we don't often exercise for. Use this challenge to improve the health of your sex life and the health of your sexual organs. It has been said that an orgasm is equivalent to running 5 miles; therefore, it is not just your sexual health that you can improve.

Sexercise

It is becoming common knowledge that sex is good exercise. Not only is it good for your body, but also for your mind, immunity and your relationship. We know that there are amazing chemicals released during sex to help us in many ways. Sex can also connect you in a spiritual nature, blending the energy of both partners together. With all the great benefits of sex it is amazing that we are still seeing couples that are having problems with it.

Sex is a great exercise and amazingly healthy for us, but it's not going to help you drop that unwanted ten pounds or so that you are carrying around. That, my friend, is going to take a little more work than just making love to your partner. Dedication to exercise (other than sex), eating right and performing mind relaxation are crucial to having an overall healthy body. Intimate play with your partner can be part of that balance.

This challenge will be a real chance for the two of you to work together and become lean, fit and mentally "on the ball". Enough chit chat - dust off your weights, unroll your yoga mat, and clear your mind. Sexercise is here.

Where to perform:

This challenge will happen in various places around your house or in your neighborhood. The intimate part of it will happen in your bedroom, but the other parts could have you running down the street, lifting weights in the basement, or finding a nice quiet corner to focus inward. You will even be in the kitchen during part of this challenge.

What you will need:

You will need any exercise equipment you love to use. This is your choice because I want you to look forward to the events to come. If bike riding is your thing, get the bike out. If meditation is your focus, then find a nice meditation mat. You will need healthy foods too. All of these choices are yours to make and agree upon as a couple. You will also need any items that you would use during your normal sexual activity. The last thing I suggest are some index cards (for the sexy part of the challenge) and a notebook where you can record your progress.

How to complete:

This challenge will gradually start moving you towards a healthier lifestyle. Jumping into radical changes is great for some people, but a gradual shift often tends to help people stick with the changes. The first thing both of you need to do is write down one healthy activity that you would like to complete each day. You can use a calendar if you wish. Some of these should be things you can do together like taking a long walk or bike riding. The others are things that you would like to do on your own. Things such as meditation or lifting weights are good choices. However, these are totally up to the each of you. Pick what you enjoy. You also need to start finding dates to change your eating habits. Pick one day a week to be vegetarian if you are not already or pick a day where you only eat fruit. (You may choose to consult with your doctor prior to changing your diet.) Do this just one day a week unless you enjoy it and then start doing it more often. Always be sure to get all of the nutrients your body needs though. Now you have a healthy plan on paper, but what about the sexy part of this challenge?

Here comes the fun part. Each of you writes on an index card a special sexual treat you would like to enjoy. It can be an interesting position, maybe the use of a toy, or maybe an intimate encounter in the shower. The only caution I suggest here is to not put things down that your partner is uncomfortable with. You might even put down a second choice as a back up. Don't show this card to your partner. Instead, seal it in an envelope and both of you put yours under the mattress of your bed.

Each day or night you both need to sit down and check off your get-healthy-plan you created earlier. Ask your partner, "Did you lift weights today?" (or whatever is on his/her list). If he/she did, give him/her a check on that day. If not, put an X. Do this each and every day of the week. Then at the end of seven days count up the checks. If your partner has achieved five checks, then he/she gets to present you with his/her envelope. At that point it is your way to honor your partner for the great work by giving him/her the sexual experience that is on the card. If you don't like the first option, then explain why to your partner and move to the second. If all goes well, you will be getting your sexual wishes and getting healthy all at the same time.

If you want to make love any other time, please do. There is no stipulation that you wait seven days to see if you have enough checks. I want to lead you to a healthy and sexually happy life. Getting into this habit you will soon find that both of you are getting into better shape. This will lead to looking better and feeling better so your sex life will improve also. What a great circle this becomes as you travel down this path of sexercise.

During this challenge think outside the box a bit and try different things. Have you ever tried yoga? What about Tai Chi? Maybe a walking meditation in a labyrinth would be a great exercise for your mind and spirit. Crossword or mind puzzles might not seem like an exercise, but research has shown that it is vital that we exercise our minds too. In fact, did you realize that the brain is actually considered an erogenous zone? You will be amazed at the different ways you can improve your health once you start looking around. Remember, I recommend that you get the okay from your doctor or healer before trying something new.

Lovers' Lane

The words "Lovers' Lane" just seem to take us back a few steps to a time when life wasn't so rushed. Imagine when young lovers would venture out with their dates and try to find a place where they could make-out. This was well before the time of computers, cell phones, etc. that keep us entertained nowadays. Back then, instead of being connected, we looked for ways to get away from the crowd and find a quiet little place for romance.

Many towns back in the fifties or sixties had places where the youth would frequent to have quiet time with their lover. Thus, the name, Lovers' Lane, was attached to many of these places. If you watch any movie from that time period, you will see that they just parked their car in the area and the focus was on kissing or whatever else could possibly happen.

This challenge is about bringing back that way of disconnecting with society and putting the focus on your lover and your lover alone. Today, it is more difficult to find a place that you can totally be alone with your lover. Plus, if you get caught making out or making love in public you are going to get a fine and possibly be humiliated by others finding out. So, how can you experience the feeling of Lovers' Lane without the risk? That is the point of this challenge.

Where to perform:

This challenge is going to happen in your car. Hopefully, you don't have a compact car. If you have more than one car, make sure to pick the one with the most room.

What you will need:

You will need all your normal supplies you have for sexual intimacy. Birth control, lube, toys, etc. can be put in a bag and placed in an easy-to-reach location within the car. Throwing some blankets into the back seat for cover and warmth is a good idea too. Towels would be nice to have around for cleanup afterwards. Music is an option you might want to bring - just make sure it is a kind that both of you enjoy.

How to complete:

Find a place to park the car where it will not get any attention. It might even be inside your garage (Just remember not to have it running with the garage door shut! That is deadly!). If you have your own property, drive out into your back yard. The beauty of the moon can have a huge romantic effect. If for some reason you cannot possibly find a secluded spot to park your car or you don't have a garage, then an option would be to set up a make believe car in your home. Place a couple of dinning room chairs in front of your couch to simulate a car. Cover the chairs with blankets so they feel more like the seats of a car.

Invite your partner to join you on a moonlit (if possible) drive. Spend a few minutes or longer driving around your neighborhood or go out and pick up a bite to eat. Make this a date. Talk about fun and exciting things that interest you. Then when the time is right, drive to your "Lovers' Lane" spot. The partner, who is the passenger, can place his/her hand on the driver's thigh on the drive or you can touch hands or arms. As you arrive at your spot slow down and pretend that you are sneaking into your own little love nest. Try to be as quiet as you can without laughing.

Slowly, slip your arm around your partner and start with a passion filled kiss. Don't hold back. Make these kisses hot and sexy. Let your hands start to roam all over each other. For the moment, keep your hands on the outside of each other's clothes. Feel your partner's body through the fabric of his/her clothes. Moving to the back seat is the signal for things to move into a more passionate state. At this point, feel free to cover up with the covers and let your hands start to roam under the clothes. Imagine this is one of the first times you have been together. After you have experienced an exciting session of lovemaking take a few moments and just be close under the blanket. Listen to each other's hearts. Hear them and feel them beating.

Appreciate each other. Be grateful that you both were willing to do something so out-of-the-ordinary. You have created a wonderful memory to recall time and time again.

Intimate Chores

We all have chores to do day in and day out. Most people don't really enjoy doing them though. Sure, they may say they don't mind doing the dishes, but do they really *enjoy* doing them. Well, this challenge will help to change that for all of you out there.

Rewards are a great way to get things done. Think about it - when you were a child did you respond to rewards? Did you get special items for cleaning your room? What about your grades in school? Did you work harder to get an A on your report card because you would get to go out for ice cream? Then, of course, there is the whole Christmas/Santa thing – be good if you want presents.

As sad as it sounds this rewards system carried over into your adult life. One of the more obvious ways in adult life revolves around getting a promotion or a new job. More often than not people behave in a certain way that is directly related to what they will receive afterwards. Putting this into your sex life is not different than the many other ways it has affected your lives. With this in mind, you are going to make doing your chores around the house a whole lot more fun and exciting.

Where to perform:

This challenge will be performed in two different areas. The first area will be where the chore will take place. The second area will be where the reward will happen. The chore part of this challenge could happen anywhere in the house, outside or even at another location. The reward area will likely be in the most comfortable and the safest place the two of you enjoy, which is usually the bedroom.

What you will need:

The challenge is also different in the fact you might need nothing for this challenge and you might need many things. This depends on the chores and the rewards your partner will want. You will have to adjust this challenge every time you perform it. Here are a couple of examples: If the chore is to vacuum the entire house, you need a vacuum. If the reward is to offer your partner a sensual massage, you need massage oil. With that being said paper and pen are the only things you will need to get started.

How to complete:

Once you and your partner have decided on performing this challenge, the first thing you need to do is address the chores and the rewards. The way it works is one partner chooses something intimate he/she would love to do with the other partner. Partner 2 evaluates the reward and chooses a chore that he/she feels would be a good trade for this intimate choice. Sit down together and both of you make a list of fun and exciting things you would like to do with your partner. You do not need to make these all sexual. You might add in things like going to see an off-Broadway show or a sporting event. Once you have your list of pleasures down, (start with 3-5) you switch papers. Look over your partner's list of pleasures and assign a chore or action to each one of them.

After you have assigned a chore or action to each item on your partner's list, give the list back to your partner (exchange these at the same time). As long as you both agree you can consider these lists as contracts. Once the chore or action is performed the other partner needs to uphold his/her part of the bargain and deliver the reward.

This can really get fun and exciting for the two of you, plus it will get some things done that might not have gotten done otherwise. Be creative with both areas and make it fun. Don't make the chores or actions impossible to perform. If your partner puts a pleasure on his/her list that you are uncomfortable with, you need to let him/her know so that another pleasure or reward can be selected.

You can also use this challenge to help out your community or Earth as a whole. You can attach chores like volunteering at your local humane society, spending a day working with Habitat for Humanity or helping clean up a local park. Any volunteer organization would love to have the help, and they don't have to know that you are getting a pleasure-filled reward for the action. It is true you have agreed for a pleasurable reward with your partner, but you will also get the emotional reward of doing something beautiful and exceptionally important.

Below is a list of suggestions of both pleasures and rewards. Of course, these are just suggestions. Your list will most likely be quite different. Once you both have completed the chores and pleasures you can start over. If you like, you can set a time limit on the contract to get things rolling a little faster.

Sample of Pleasures / Chores (actions)
1. Make love in shower / Scrub and clean entire bathroom
2. Sensual massage / Clean windows on outside
3. Oral sex / Clean out the garage
4. Try a new position / Fold and put away all laundry
5. Let partner blindfold you / 4 hours volunteering at homeless shelter
6. Tickets to sporting event or concert/ Paint outside of house
7. Sex ten days in a row / Cooking dinner ten days in a row
8. Wear something sexy / Take out the trash

This challenge can be a fun and wonderful way for partners to connect. Yet, **do not make all of your intimacy a reward for a chore**. If you ever find yourself saying, "Well I am not making love to you until you do (a specific chore)," then you have gone too far!! This challenge is meant to just be a little extra way to appreciate your partner - not belittle or control him/her. Always use it in a loving manner.

Shower Magick

Most of the people in the world today have a desire to be clean. Even those people in areas that do not have the luxury of indoor plumbing will still venture down to the local stream to bathe. This refreshing feeling of washing the dirt off of your body is one of those enjoyable parts of life. The feeling you get as that water first hits you from your shower or as you slowly submerge your body into a warm bathtub is truly magickal. (This is special magick – so it is spelled with a "k".)

Even as wonderful and sensual as showers and baths can be we still don't enjoy them with our partner very often. Bathing has become a morning or evening ritual for most people - just to get clean. It is usually just a jump in the shower get clean and head off to work. As with all good things, we need to sometimes slow down and share this enjoyment with the one we love.

Incorporating your beloved into a shower or bath with you isn't something that normally just happens. It takes planning and effort. First of all, you have to get comfortable sharing this space with your partner. Typically, you reserve this space and time just for yourself. Therefore, you need to prepare to adjust your intention. Wrap your mind around the idea of sharing the space. This new intention can create a magickal energy in and around your shower.

This experience is going to show you and your lover how to change up your normal bathing routine. It will show you how to be present with your beloved while enjoying the warm and passionate water that surrounds you both. It will allow your passion to flow freely and openly to express the love that you feel. Just as the rain helps bring forth the flowers, the water flowing around us can bring forth love.

Where to perform:

This challenge will obviously take place in your shower or bathtub. It might move on to other areas of your home, but the focus is on what goes on in the bathing area.

What you will need:

You will need two to four of the biggest softest towels you have. If you don't have any, go out and purchase them as a special treat. Next, I suggest getting different soaps and shampoos than you normally use. Get ones with a distinctive smell to them so that the two of you will start to associate the scent with your shower magick. Put these items away after you are done with this challenge. Keep them unique to this bathing ritual instead of allowing them to become mundane with everyday use. Bring them out whenever you want to enjoy this challenge again. Other items I suggest include candles (I always suggest the flameless ones for safety), music, wash clothes, and maybe even a little wine. If you are going to take a bath, you could also bring an erotic story to read to each other and possibly even finger foods. Be creative and bring items that might heighten sensations as you clean each other. Sponges, loofas, or a back scrubber can all add excitement to the enjoyment of the water and this experience.

How to complete:

The first thing you must do is get everything purchased that you need. Items like the soaps, towels, wine, etc. must be on hand. Once you have these items your first objective is to invite your beloved partner to come and enjoy the bath or shower with you. Then the magickal bathing can begin. I will address baths and showers separately as they demand different attention.

If you and your lover a going to take a magickal bath together then you need to fill the tub with warm water. Both of you should test the water making sure it is a wonderful temperature for each of you. Lay your fluffy towels within easy reach for when you exit your bath. Place all the other items within reach of the bathtub. (Remember – though this should be obvious – to keep any electrical items, such as stereos, away from the tub.) Add scented oils or bath salts to the water. This makes the water come to life. Turn on a little soft background music. Turn the lights down, and let the candles be your only source of light. Once all things are in place it is time for both of you to enter the water.

In the bathtub, you can sit either face to face or one behind the other. Take time and wash each other. It is not necessary to focus on cleaning. Instead, allowing the water run over your body can be a wondrous sensation. Make it a point to feel your partner's body while it is slick with water. Spend some time just caressing each other. You can even explore your partner's body with your feet too. Relax and enjoy the warm water and quiet time with your lover. If you have some erotic stories, this would be a good time to read them to each other. If you brought wine and/or finger foods, enjoy them now as well. Most importantly look deep into your partner's eyes and express your love without speaking a word - let your eyes say, "I love you."

For a different way to experience a magickal bath, turn out all of the lights and enjoy the bath and the presence of your lover in total darkness. Allow your hands to touch each other as a substitute for your vision. You could also make love in the bathtub.

Once you are finished, take turns drying each other off. Use more of a patting method than rubbing. If your clothes dryer is in your bathing area or if you have a small heater, you can have your towels warmed-up for when you get out of the water.

Now, for those of you who will be showering instead, start out the same with getting everything in place and the music playing. See how close the two of you can get allowing your hands to explore each other's backsides. This will help keep both of you under the warm spray. Massage shampoo into each other's hair and let the gentle rain of the shower wash all your cares away. Bring your wine glasses into the shower if you have room. The glasses may get a bit slippery in the steam; therefore, be careful not to drop them. Take turns turning around to allow your partner to wash your back as never before. There are advantages to having a helping hand in the shower. Turn all the lights out while the two of you are in the shower and let your hands light the way.

You can, also, make love in the shower and enjoy the caressing water as your bodies become one. Kiss passionately under the cascade of water. Splash around and watch how the water trickles down the curves of your lover's body. Be present with all your attention and enjoy the moment and memories you are creating. Once you are finished get your big soft towels (heated if the dryer is near the shower area) and pat each other dry as you look deep into your partner's eyes. End with a passionate kiss and a long embrace.

After either of these activities you can move the action to other areas of the house to keep the passion going. Other options you might consider would be bringing some toys into the shower to experiment with. You could float flower petals in the water or fill the tub with as many rubber ducks as you can find. Do your best to make this time a memorable occasion. The next time you take your normal shower or bath you will likely have a little smile of pleasure upon your face and in your heart.

Heart Shaped Box

Expressing your desires to your partner is sometimes hard to do. Sometimes it is easier to just show him/her. In this challenge, I will show you a way to get your point across without having to verbalize it.

Communication is not always speaking to one another. You have several other ways to communicate. Some people can write out what they want to say much better than just speaking the words. While others take a more visual approach to communication, such as painting or building sculptures to communicate their feelings to the world. You may have a favorite way of communicating or excel in a particular way, but you shouldn't judge those that cannot communicate in the same way. Simply telling your partner to speak what is on his/her mind isn't always the answer. If this is not the way your partner communicates, you cannot expect him/her to just change and open up by talking simply because you want or expect it.

Once you find the best way for the two of you to communicate things will start to flow in a much better manner. It is important to know that you don't have to stick with one form of communication. Sometimes people can use different communication skills for different situations. For example, someone might be able to talk freely and openly about the finances of your relationship, but when it comes to the intimacy in your relationship he/she clams up. The heart shaped box is a different way to connect. You can learn to use it in many areas of your relationship.

Where to perform:

This challenge can be performed any place and at any time. Privacy is the only thing you will really need. You don't want others to witness what you might discover about your lover. Plus, this information is for your eyes only and even an unsuspecting witness could take away from this joy between the two of you.

What you will need:

Find a heart shaped box – these are often easier to find around Valentine's Day. If you can't find a heart shaped box, you can use another type of box. However, I suggest you decorate it with hearts or images that convey love. Make sure your box is a pretty good size. Some of the things you and your partner will put in the box are larger items.

How to complete:

This box is going to be a communication portal for your relationship. It is just one way of communication – so keep talking to each other and communicating in other ways too. This particular challenge is a new way to communicate about your intimate life, but you can use it for other areas of your relationship too.

Hide your box out of view from others as its contents should only be shared between the two of you. Place it in a drawer or on a special shelf in your closet. Make a ceremony out of checking its contents each and every week. Agree on a special time once a week that each of you will go through the contents and add your own. Do this separately from one another. Select different days for each of you so that you have time to respond and/or add another item.

You can put anything you desire into the box that will be of interest to your partner and you. You can put items in the box or even questions for your lover. You can even go so far as to place a new toy or new bottle of oil in the box – if this is something you would like to try with your partner. Tickets to a show or a note about dinner reservations work well too. Other items might include pictures from special occasions, vacation ideas, a poem for your love, a book, an article on aphrodisiacs, lingerie, etc. The object is to create a free flowing means of conversing about intimacy and passion in a romantic way.

If your partner puts something in the box that you are uncomfortable with or refuse to try, explain this to him/her in another box entry. It is helpful if you try to explain why instead of just refusing, but it is important to at least let your partner know that you are uncomfortable even if you don't fully understand why yourself. Also, be aware that just because you put the item in the box doesn't mean it will get used or be part of your intimacy. The point is to start freely communicating things you would love to have in your relationship (emotionally and physically). It might be something as simple as snuggling more or as complex as full out role-playing.

Honor your partner and your relationship by staying on schedule. When it is your day to check the contents – do so. If something happens and you are unable to check on your scheduled day, let your partner know and make appropriate adjustments. See if you can keep the secret and the excitement of the Heart Shaped Box going for as long as you need. Perhaps, at some point it will be just a metaphor the two of you will use to make it known that you have wishes, passionate dreams, or desires you want to discuss.

Hot and Cold

Nothing changes our sensations like switching from one extreme to the other. Here is one example: try doing something in the dark that you would normally do in the light - maybe picking out your clothes. You have to use a whole different process than when your room is lit up with that magical thing we call light. In the dark, you use other senses to compensate for your lack of sight.

In this challenge, you are going to use two extremes to change the level of excitement in your intimacy. Those extremes are "hot" and "cold". One can make you sweat and strip your clothes off and the other can make you shiver from head to toe and put on as many clothes as you can. These are the two temperatures that everyone complains about. You hear people say, "It's too Hot!" or "It's too cold!" Yet, it is highly unlikely that you will you hear anyone say, "It's too lukewarm".

How can hitting both extremes be sexy? That is where I am going to take you. So get prepared to experience intimacy so hot it makes you sweat and in the same fashion intimacy so cold it will send shivers down your spine. Both of these will make you feel vibrant and alive with passion. This challenge could actually unite the sunbathers near the equator with the polar bear clubs of the north into one community. Get out your sunscreen and your mittens, for you will need both.

Where to perform:

This challenge needs to take place where you can produce both hot and cold experiences for your partner. You could rent a hotel room, but you can also do this at home where everything is at your fingertips. Plus who knows how you are going to react to the extremes. You might scream out with pleasure and personally I think it would be better to do that at home. However, the choice is up to you and your partner.

What you will need:

There are so many things you could bring into this challenge that I could not possibly name all of them. I will suggest a few here, but feel free to branch out and bring things that you feel would work well. Ice cube trays, bottled water, cups, heating pads, cold packs, hand warmers, eye droppers, big fluffy towels, warm sheets, fans, electric heaters, and firewood are a few items that come to mind. Sex toys and lube are other items you may want. Also, if you use birth control or other safe sex items such as condoms, bring them too.

How to complete:

Start off by taking a shower. If your shower is big enough for the two of you, then share your shower. If not, you can go one at a time. Of course, sharing is so much more fun. Turn the water on as hot as you are both comfortable with. Enjoy the warming sensation as it opens up your pours and relaxes you. Then quickly turn the water to a much colder setting. See how your body reacts to the extreme of cold. After a moment or two turn the water back to warm and let your body enjoy opening back up to the heat of the shower. Do this as often as you like and witness how your body adjusts going from hot to cold to hot again. Once you are done with your shower, get your big fluffy towels and dry yourselves off. But, don't stay snuggled up in your warm towels. Instead, drop them and streak to the bed. To add more excitement to this, turn on some fans or turn up the air conditioning before you get into the shower. This will create a much colder space to streak through. Dive under the covers and warm each other up.

Now, you can move on to some more intimate play with your new friends hot and cold. You might even consider pointing your fans toward your bed. Start out by kissing each other under the covers. Then one of you throw the covers off and let the cool air of the fan chill your bodies as you are still passionately kissing. Then without stopping the kissing the other partner reaches down and pulls the covers back up to warm your bodies. Wait at least ten seconds before reaching for the covers.

Move on to some more intimate foreplay bringing the hot and cold to your erogenous zones. Start with your cold packs and hand warmer packs. Break them both to start the reaction and place the cold pack on an erotic area of your partner. If he/she can stand it, wait about five to ten seconds then switch it out for the heat pack. Take turns doing this back and forth for as long as you like. Make sure to hit areas such as the nipples, breasts, testicles, and labia as well as areas such as the feet, underarms, neck and small of the back. Hopefully, you know your partner well enough to know the areas that turn him/her on. You can also fill up a couple of cups of water putting ice cubes in one and heating the other up. Use an eyedropper to gently let the water drip on your partner switching back and forth from cold to hot. For added excitement, blindfold your partner – this will prevent him/her from knowing what to expect – hot or cold.

Now, experiment with the genitals. The first way you are going to do this is by performing oral sex on your partner. First get a nice cold drink or even put some ice in your mouth to give your partner a frosty oral sensation. After sharing the coldness of your lips and tongue on your partner take a drink of something hot (don't burn your mouth) such as tea.

Continue your kissing and oral loving with a hot mouth. This switch from cold to hot and perhaps back again is a sensation that everyone should experience at least once in his/her sexual lifetime. You can also use the hot and cold liquids to warm up or cool down your sex toys. Oohhhh my! This could possibly be one of the most exciting experiences your lover has ever enjoyed. The experience of switching back and forth between extremes will have your lover begging for more and more and more.

One final thought I would like to share is the idea of using snow. If you happen to have snow in your area, bring some in and use it to excite your lover. You could do this in front of a roaring fireplace – how romantic.

CAUTION: Make sure your items are not too hot or too cold. The intention is not for either of you to be harmed. This challenge is to help you tantalize each other. Test all items out before placing them on your partner and stop immediately if you partner seems to be in discomfort.

All Day Arousal

One of the best parts of any sexual experience is getting aroused. The feeling that creeps over you as your blood starts pumping is one of the simple joys in life. The problems lies in that sometimes, much like the orgasm, it is over way too quickly. Now, as for orgasms, there are not many ways to stretch them out. Arousal, however, is a little more under your control whether you are the one that is arousing your partner or the one being aroused.

This challenge is not only going to test you, but it is going to extend your arousal all day long. Using these little tips and suggestions you and your partner will greatly anticipate the moment when you can finally find the time to enjoy all this arousal you have been experiencing. This anticipation will make the results so much sweeter and even more passionate. Think about the last time you had to wait for something and how much better it made it. When you finally got what you were waiting on didn't you savor it that much more?

Both of you are in control of this challenge and you both are going to reap the benefits. Anticipation and excitement are not only great things to experience, but they can be good for your health. They get your heart pumping and your mind working as you imagine how great things will be. Your intention will bring you amazing experiences because you are focusing on them.

What you will need:

Wow, where to begin with what you need for this challenge? It will be hard to cover everything. So, I am going to tell you right now to branch out and use any means possible to arouse your partner. You can send an email, text or video and with modern technology your partner can receive this instantly. (*Remember to use your discretion when creating videos or pictures.) So, cameras, computers, and phones are all important things to have around. Paper and pen for writing notes is a good thing to have for this challenge, too. The basic principal of what you need is anything that can convey an intimate message to your partner. The possibilities are endless, however the more imaginative you are the better.

Where to perform:

This challenge will happen anywhere that both of you will be during the day. It will start in the morning as you are getting ready for work, follow you to work, be with you at lunch, on the ride home and eventually when you meet up later to let the emotions of the arousal release within the both of you. This challenge may take a lot of planning to make everything work out, but will be well worth it.

How to complete:

The object is to keep your partner aroused all day long. This does not mean he/she will be physically aroused all day. Instead, it will shift from physical to emotional to mental and back to physical. Your goal is to find ways that will keep your partner anticipating physical intimacy with you later toward the end of the day. Let me give you some ideas on how to accomplish this.

Planning is the key. You cannot go into this challenge and just expect it to happen. It is important to plan. Start in the morning and think through his/her routine. What can you add to his/her daily morning activities that will bring about sensual thoughts of you? Consider your partner's whole day. Then start looking for areas to slip in your little mental reminder of the passion you wish to share later in the day.

- You could start in the bathroom with a note on the mirror. Tell your partner how sexy he/she looks in pajamas.
- You could put a note on the shampoo expressing how you are going to run your fingers through his/her hair later that evening.

- Put a note in his/her brief case mentioning something sexy you are going to do to after you both get home.
- You might slip a sexy pair of underwear in the pocket of his/her jacket.
- You could put a gift certificate to a special restaurant on the seat of his/her car with instructions for dinner later.
- You could plan out sexy text or email messages to your beloved while he/she is at work.
- Another interesting thing to do would be to take a picture of a part of your body and put it where your partner will find it. For ladies a picture of your legs with a note attached saying something sexy or for men maybe you take a picture of your flexed muscles and attach a note telling your partner you can't wait to get your arms around him/her.

Some other ideas include: leave sexy phone messages, hide all the normal sleepwear and replace it with sexier items, or pay for him/her to get a therapeutic massage at the spa to get those muscles all loosened up.

Continue this stimulation throughout the day, without over doing it. You may only want to do two or three of these things within any given day. Too many items like this might get annoying. Again, be sure to use discretion – inappropriate messages, pictures, or actions at your partner's work could be embarrassing or even get your partner in trouble.

When you get home you can continue with more. One great thing to do is to meet your love at home with the most passionate kiss you can muster. You don't have to meet at the door unless it just works out, but you could lay this juicy kiss on him/her right before you two begin eating dinner. Being in the privacy of your home you can increase the sexiness of your attention. Touch your partner in sexy ways. Slide your hand across the small of her back or run your hand down the front of his chest. Remember this is about anticipation.

Maybe you can find a sensual movie for the two of you to watch or play a game with a sexy theme. Leave sexy things lying around for your beloved to find. Start a sexy conversation. You might leave a pair of your panties on the computer or position a sex toy by his/her toothbrush. Draw this out until you feel you have pushed it as far as you can. Then at that moment, find your partner, grab him/her by the hand and head to the bedroom. Slam the door shut and proceed to make passionate love. Don't hold anything back.

You don't need to do this for each other on the same day. If necessary, take turns. Giving and receiving are both amazing feelings. Most likely, you love to be the object of your partner's affection, but it is just as amazing to be the one that is turning up the heat. Don't be shy. Use your imagination. It makes it that much more memorable.

Dodge Ball

It seems to me that dodge ball is one of the most senseless games ever created. Throwing a ball and trying to hit opponents in any way is not only brutal, but only caters to the stronger and more agile people. These life skills are not as vital for survival as they once were. Being able to chuck a ball the hardest in no way shape or form can help you succeed in business unless you are an NFL Quarterback. Being quick enough to dodge a speeding ball typically doesn't come in handy in our modern society either. So, other than power and speed what can you get out of dodge ball? Well, it can be a lot of fun.

This version of dodge ball is a little different. Instead of trying to physically harm each other during the course of the game you are going to use the basic premise of the game to put more passion and love into your relationship. How can you throw things at each other and get a positive response out of it? Well, I have an idea. Keep reading to find out, and soon you will be asking your lover if he/she would like to play a game of dodge ball with you. This request will have your partner jumping out of the chair to do so.

Most dodge ball games consist of teams of players. This version is a more intimate game and should be played between just two players. In this version, getting hit is just as much fun as being the person who is doing the throwing. Both of you will become love targets. Who would have ever guessed that dodge ball could become a form of foreplay? Sound exciting? Well, you better warm up and get ready to dodge and love your way to fun.

What you will need:

You will need soft balls to throw. Foam balls from the toy department of your local discount store work well. I suggest you use ones that are the size of a softball or smaller. They should be just big enough to easily wrap your hand around. If you don't want to purchase any items, you could take several pairs of socks and roll them up inside each other to form a ball. Have at least three balls for each participant. You will need one towel for each player as well. These will be used to set your playing zone.

Where to perform:

You need to perform this in an open space. You should be at least 10 feet apart and away from anything that might be breakable. Look closely at the area and remove anything that might be affected by a ball hitting it. Items like picture frames, lamps, or trinkets should be moved away from the playing area. Also, play this in a place that both of you can be naked. As often is the case, your bedroom might end up being the best place for your challenge.

How to complete:

Decide upon the distance between your playing zones. When deciding this take into account the balls you will be using. The foam balls are hard to throw a great distance, while rolled up socks can be thrown longer distances with no trouble. Once you both agree on the distance you need to lay your towels on the floor that far apart. (Be cautious if you have non-carpeted floors as the towels might be slippery on the floor.) Yoga mats make a great substitute for the towels if you have them. The area of your towel is your personal play area. You both have to stay on your towel. The only reason to leave the towel is to retrieve the balls.

Start out the game fully clothed. Divide up the balls evenly between the players. Once each player is on his/her mat/towel the game can begin. As in the original dodge ball game the object is to strike your partner with the ball. However, the result of being struck does not produce the same outcome. When a player is struck in an area he/she must remove the clothing upon that area. If the first person hits you in the leg you must remove your pants. If you are hit in the chest, stomach, arm, or back you must remove your shirt, etc. The game continues until one player is completely naked. The player that still has clothing on is the victor and gets to proceed to the winner's circle.

In the winners circle the victor is allowed to ask for special attention during this night's sexual activity. He/she may request oral sex, a massage, extra foreplay, or anything that is agreed upon by both of you. You might want to agree upon a number of requests for the victor before the game starts to avoid confusion during this time. Experiencing an ending ceremony to your dodge ball festivities can be great fun.

Important notes: There are several variables that the partners will have to agree upon before the game starts. For starters, is the throwing just a free for all or do you take turns chucking the balls at each other. You also need to decide when it is okay to leave your playing area to retrieve more ammo (balls in this case). Can you do this as soon as you run out of balls or do you need to wait until both partners are out of balls? You need to decide what happens if you are struck in an area that already had the clothing removed. Does the striker get to choose another piece of clothing to remove or does the one that has been struck get to choose. Or is that hit simply null and void? You could go in a different direction and agree that if you are struck in an area that doesn't have any clothing, the opponent gets to kiss the area stuck.

Will you only allow direct hits or can the ball bounce off of things like walls, floor or the ceiling? You might want to set a number of clothing items to wear in the beginning so that each partner has the same amount of items on. Then what penalties will you put into place for falling off or leaving the playing area? You could say leaving the towel or mat costs that participant one item of clothing or you could have penalty shots where the other partner gets all the balls and gets to throw them.

This challenge can be loads of fun, but always remember safety. If you are in your socks, remember the floor might be slippery off of your playing area. If you wear glasses or jewelry, you may want to remove them to avoid injury. Make sure to use any methods of safe sex you would normally use. Most importantly enjoy a good laugh with your partner and share a new kind of intimate play.

OOOOOOOHHH! Christmas Tree

Christmas time rolls around and our thoughts change to those of spreading love and creating good will on Earth. At least, we hope those are what your thoughts change to. Not everyone celebrates Christmas, but you can adjust this challenge to accommodate any religion or belief system.

The beauty of Christmas to me is the special feeling that you get from expressing your love to those you care about the most. The world itself seems to become a little friendlier at this time of year – in general anyway. You are going to take this passion the world has and use it to spread even more love and intimacy into your relationship.

I am going to give you a couple of different scenarios that you can use to create joy in your relationship during this time of year. Showering each other with the passion and love of the season is a great way to show each other how truly special you are to one another. You don't have to use this challenge only during the holiday season. Feel free you to adjust it for birthdays, anniversaries, or any other special day or holiday you might want to celebrate. Showing your beloved that he/she is the object of your affection is the point you are trying to make. You are getting ready to celebrate the holidays in the most jolly of ways.

What you will need:

The most important thing you will need for this challenge is a small Christmas tree. It can be an artificial one or a real one. You will also need decorations for it, such as ornaments, lights, or handcrafted things to place upon your tree. The gifts you will give to your partner during this challenge can be purchased from a store or they can be homemade. One homemade gift idea is to make up "coupons" or "gift certificates" for things like back rubs, a night out for dinner and a movie, a bottle of his/her favorite wine, doing your partner's chores for him/her etc. You will need some of your favorite festive music. An iPod, computer, CD player all work well for this. You can also find radio stations that only play Christmas music at this time of year. I encourage you to be creative and tailor all the items to you and your partner. This is your experience and no one else's.

Where to perform:

If it is just the two of you in the house during the holidays, you can place your special tree and decorations anywhere you would like. If you have little children, you will have to keep your tree in a place out of reach and away from the normal traffic area in your home. Your bedroom is a great place. It is important to take into consideration that you may have items around your tree that are private and should only be shared between the two of you. If you don't have the space for a tree in your home, you could always get a special plant to serve the purpose. A few options are Poinsettias, small ferns, or a Christmas cactus. (Remember some plants can be poisonous to pets and children – or at least cause upset stomachs or rashes.)

How to complete:

Begin this challenge around the first of December. This will give you and your love plenty of time to enjoy the OOOOOHHHH Christmas Tree. The tree that you are going to put up during this challenge is dedicated to your intimate passion and love for each other. It will serve as a reminder during this holiday season of how sexy your relationship can be. Choose a time to spend a little while together setting up your space with this tree of passion. Make it a ceremony and maybe even an annual ritual for the two of you. Once you have the tree set up, you can decide how you want to proceed.

The first choice is to surround the tree with intimate presents for each other. These types of presents might include things like sex toys, lubes, intimate apparel and coupons for intimate favors for your lover. These are placed under your tree-of-love as gifts for your beloved. Just like ordinary presents they sit there and wait for Christmas Day to be opened. You might have to wait for Christmas night or you can get an early start on the holiday and give each other these special gifts on Christmas Eve. You could also give your lover a present from under this tree on the days leading up to Christmas. Maybe you both make a pact that you get twelve intimate presents and have your own special twelve days of Christmas celebration. This way of celebrating your love at Christmas fits with the way many people celebrate the holidays.

Here are some different ideas to complete this challenge. One suggestion would be to not put any decorations on the tree after setting it up. Then each time leading up to Christmas that you make love or have an intimate experience you place an ornament on the tree. See how full you can make your tree. If you would like to carry this challenge over to next Christmas, count the number of ornaments you added to the tree after Christmas has passed. Write this down somewhere you will be able to find again next year. Then do this challenge again next year. You will be able to compare the number of ornaments against each one other.

Another great option is to use intimate apparel, toys or condoms as decorations for your tree. Make it a priority to wear or use each and every item hanging on the tree or around the room before Christmas. Some examples of apparel might be really sexy stockings hanging from the mantle or as garland on your small tree (Nookies

Pleasure Sox work well here), or sex toys or condoms hung on the tree like ornaments. You could even add paper ornaments with names of sexy Christmas songs to play during your lovemaking or with suggestions of things you would like to do during lovemaking.

The best part of this challenge is bringing romance back to the holidays. I don't want you to compete against one another, but you might try to add something else every time your partner adds something. There are no losers, you both win and win big. Your Christmas or holidays will never be the same again. I hope you turn this into an annual tradition for the two of you.

New Year's Resolution

Every year we go through the same old resolutions. We are going to lose weight, stop smoking, and be more environmentally conscious, just to name a few. They are all great and important to the health of our bodies and our environment. However, most of these New Year's Resolutions fall flat. Why, does it happen? Why can we not stick to our resolutions and make the changes we want to make?

Well, most of the time it is because we don't have the support system in place. It's not that we don't have the dedication to follow through. I believe that most of us fail because we are the only person rooting for us to uphold our New Year's resolutions. If we had an outside source rooting for us and helping track our progress, or lifting us up when we are down, things might be a little different.

That is the concept of this challenge. You are going to be support for each other in the pursuit of keeping your New Year's resolution in tact. You are going to be the coach urging your partner on to reach that goal and change his/her lifestyle. Improvement is the goal and you will stand together as you near it. Now, to put an intimate feel into this New Year's Resolution, I am going to share with you another option.

Your focus for this New Year will be to improve the quality, quantity and power in your sexual relationship. This will allow both partners to create and experience the joy and passion that finding your sexual groove will bring. It is always easy to push things off and work on them later, but not today. I want you both to make a commitment to become super lovers with each other.

My goal is to create the most passionate and magical relationships in the world. I hope that each couple I help find their blended spirit will spread the message and help other couples. I want to shift the world into a more passionate and loving place. Thank you for taking the time to get involved in this challenge. I am honored to be a part of your lives via this medium.

Where to perform:

You can do this challenge anywhere as it takes on a life of it's own and moves freely from place to place this coming year. One of the goals of this challenge is to spark new and exciting ways to be intimate. Venturing outside of your normal lovemaking areas might be something you add to your sexy New Year's resolution.

What you will need:

What you need will depend on how you set up your New Year's resolution. Are you going to want to try new things, new toys, or new adventures in lovemaking? If so, you will have to plan on getting the items necessary to achieve these goals. If you want to try a little light bondage this coming year, you will need items to achieve that. If you want to make love in France, you will probably need plane tickets and passports. The pure beauty of this is that it is going to be totally built for the two of you. The items needed will be a clear indication of where you will lead this challenge.

How to complete:

Okay, I have lots of ground to cover in building your challenge. Your first option has to do with the quantity of intimate play you will have in the coming year. Many people might think it crazy to keep track of how many times you make love in a year, but why be like most people? Try to get an idea of how many times in the last year you made love. If you made love once a week, then 52 would be a good guess. If it happened once a month, then 12 times (yikes) a year would be your answer. I want you to set your goal a little higher, but within reason. Shooting for 365 times a year is a bit unrealistic. I suggest trying to reach 100. This will average out to be 8 times a month with 4 bonus ones sometime throughout the year.

Once you have your amount set then make a chart to keep track. Get stickers to place on a calendar or keep a tote board over your bed if you really want to be silly. Part of the fun is to celebrate when you hit milestones. Make it a little more special when you hit number 25, 50, 75 etc. When you start nearing your goal for the year plan out a bigger celebration - maybe a fancy dinner at a nice restaurant or a trip to a special location. Plan whatever suits the two of you best. You might even want to plan it out so your magical number is performed on a vacation or in a fancy hotel. All these options are up to the two of you. Just make a point to make it a special occasion. You don't have to shoot off fireworks, but don't let it pass without acknowledgement.

Another option might be to make a point to try something different sexually in the upcoming year. Select several different things to make the resolution last longer. If you want to be really creative, pick an exciting activity for each month. If you only pick one, it could be over on New Year's Day and I want you to enjoy throughout your entire year. One thing that might help you with this option is to check out a classy company that sells sexual items – toys, oils, etc. You can visit a brick-and-mortar store or you can check some out online. Go through their items together and make a list of ones that interest the two of you. You can also find things you haven't tried before instead of picking out an item. For example, some couples have never tried oral sex, so that could be a choice for them. Heck it might even be a different location in your house such as the shower or in the recliner. Be open to the idea, but if your partner says, "NO WAY!" ditch it and pick again.

Here are a list of some things you might consider: Lingerie or intimate apparel, light bondage items, different types of lubrication, different locations in the house, oral sex, anal sex, mutual masturbation, body paints, food items eaten off each other, role playing, or doing a different sexy challenge each month. The list could go on and on, but you get the idea. Set your list and then set your sexy New Year's resolution in motion. You might just find yourself learning that you like some of these things enough where they become part of your normal intimate play.

I have one last option for you, but this one truly takes some planning. In this option, you agree to try and make love in as many different places as you can. I am not talking about in your home. I am talking about traveling to different locations such as vacations or weekend getaways to make love. This option takes a bit more money than the others do. So, watch for deals. The location doesn't have to be far away. It could be in the next city over or even when you visit relatives. The point is to make love in as many different locations as you can this coming year.

Other options you might consider include performing sacred ceremonies (such as in the Intimate Adventures:

Sacred Ceremonies for Couples series) or honoring each other every time you are intimate with a special treat afterwards. No matter what you decide to put into your sexy New Year's resolution it will show a dedication to your lover and to your relationship. Working together on this resolution will give each of you the support you need to keep this New Year's resolution going strong for the entire year. If you can make it last the entire year, then you can revamp it for the next year. Of course, if you do not make it through the year, you can still start over and try again next year.

Bonus

Intimate Adventures

Nature Lovers

Physical intimacy is a wonderful and natural thing. We often seem to forget how connected to nature we are though. We need to remove our religious beliefs, our social beliefs, and our negative beliefs from physical intimacy. We need to honor it as it is supposed to honored. Do you always honor your partner before, during and after intimacy? Have you thought about this before?

In this intimate adventure, you are going to give him/her an offering to not only show your love, but as a way to honor the union of your intimacy. Many cultures have honored intimacy and fertility in ways that are too numerous for me to mention here. Some of these that stand out to me include the Pagan ritual where the lovers would make love in the fields to ensure that the crops would be bountiful as well as many sex magick rituals where the sexual energy is directed to help a specific area or need such as getting a new job or healing an illness. With this intimate adventure you will learn a new way to honor your relationship. The offering you are going to present your beloved and your union is a bit of nature.

To start you and your partner must both go out into nature and spend some time with no set plan or destination. It does not matter where you live. Even in a city you can encounter nature – you just have to look. When you go into nature you can either do it alone or together. If you go together, you might want to separate for a bit to keep the offering you are going to find a secret. During this time open your senses and feel what item calls to you. It might be a small rock, a flower, a stick or even a fallen leaf. No matter what the element is as you approach it carefully look around the area. See how this piece of nature is a part of its surroundings. Before you pick up this wonderful work of art nature has provided ask for permission to take it. This may seem very strange to you, but we should not just take something from nature simply because we want it. When you feel the call of something most likely you will sense that it is all right to take it with you, but still ask (you can ask quietly in your mind – no one needs to hear you). If you feel you should not take it or if it is too large to take, then take a photo instead. Thank this piece of nature in helping you honor your beloved and your union. After offering gratitude to nature take the item or the photo of the item and return home or meet back up with your partner.

Slip your object of honor into your pocket if possible to keep it hidden from your lover. **You might want to take a small bag with you in case what you find is too large to place in a pocket. Once home you may want to wash your object and make it more presentable or you may choose to leave it as it. If you feel compelled, you might add decoration like beads or feathers to the item – you might even consider painting something on it. Of course, you most certainly can leave it in its truest form. As you both now have your honor object I suggest you take a shower and cleanse your bodies. You may do this together or separate. Another wonderful thing you may choose to do is to light a candle or burn some incense. You may also consider playing music softly– something earthy or filled with sounds of nature. If you do this in a lowly lit area of your home, you can heighten your experience.

Bring your objects of honor and sit across from each other. Gently place the objects or photos between you. Take turns presenting your object to your beloved. As you pick up your item and show it to him/her say something like, "With this piece of nature I honor all that is natural between us. I honor our love and our union with this amazing work of art from nature." And, then share a powerful or wondrous quality about the item that you can relate to your partner.

Once both of you have done, this choose a place where you can set your nature items as a reminder of this honoring. You can put them on a shelf, your desk, the dining table, etc. Before placing them in this place of honor you may want to keep them around the place you make love to energize them and fill them with your passion. Keep these items for as long as you wish or for as long as is feasible. I suggest that at some point you return them to nature. This will send your intimate and love-filled energy into nature and it will deepen its connection with the Universe. Returning these objects of honor is a ritual in its own right that you should do together as a couple. If possible, I suggest you do it under the light of the moon. Create something small to say as you do this such as, "These items have honored our union and with our love we return them to nature to share our love and intimate energy with the world and the Universe for others so they may too experience their own."

This is a very profound and humbling experience to combine your intimate connection with your partner to nature. Remember that truly our need and desire for connection with one another is natural – it comes from nature – we are a part of nature. Maybe if you do this more often, you will start to feel more connected with Earth. Do this and Earth will connect more with the both of you!

Stay connected with Rob

by signing up for the Inward Oasis Newsletter at

http://sexychallenges.com

and like Sexy Challenges on Facebook

http://www.facebook.com/SexyChallengesatInwardOasis